'A tale of dispossession, displacement, and remarkable resilience. Epic in scope, but always grounded in the domestic, it chronicles one woman's struggle to live a fulfilling life, despite her blindness and lack of education. Marie Younan is an engaging storyteller: intimate, warm, direct, and honest. In Jill Sanguinetti she has a skilful writer who has worked with her to create a rich tapestry, interweaving ancient and contemporary Assyrian history and a vast gallery of family characters, teachers, friends, and support workers who have taken part in her journey.'

ARNOLD ZABLE, writer, novelist,
and human rights advocate

'Huge-hearted and inspiring.
A book that literally makes us see the world in new ways.'

CHLOE HOOPER, award-winning author of
The Tall Man and *The Arsonist*

'A story, raw with reality, full of love and hope, where the stream of resilience runs clear. We share the life of someone for whom blindness is not the insurmountable barrier many believe it to be. What most holds Marie back is the problem of low expectations. It is hard to put this book down.'

GRAEME INNES AM, former Australian Disability
Discrimination Commissioner

A DIFFERENT KIND OF SEEING

Marie Younan is an interpreter with refugees and counsellors at Foundation House — the Victorian Foundation for Survivors of Torture Inc., in Melbourne.

Jill Sanguinetti is a retired lecturer and researcher in education. Her childhood memoir, *School Days of a Methodist Lady: a journey through girlhood*, was published by Wild Dingo Press in 2014.

A DIFFERENT KIND OF SEEING

MY JOURNEY

MARIE YOUNAN

WITH JILL SANGUINETTI

SCRIBE

Melbourne • London

Scribe Publications

18–20 Edward St, Brunswick, Victoria 3056, Australia
2 John St, Clerkenwell, London, WC1N 2ES, United Kingdom
3754 Pleasant Ave, Suite 100, Minneapolis, Minnesota 55409, USA

First published by Scribe 2020
Copyright © Marie Younan and Jill Sanguinetti 2020

Typeset in Adobe Garamond Pro by the publishers

Printed and bound in Australia by Griffin Press, part of Ovato

Scribe Publications is committed to the sustainable use of natural resources and the use of paper products made responsibly from those resources.

9781922310255 (paperback edition)
9781925938616 (ebook)

A catalogue record for this book is available from the National Library of Australia.

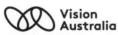

Blindness. Low Vision. Opportunity.

This publication was proudly sponsored by Vision Australia.

scribepublications.com.au
scribepublications.com

I dedicate this book to the memory of
BEN HEWITT
(1930—2014)
my braille teacher, life mentor, and friend.

•

Ben taught me how to see
— a different kind of seeing.

More than at any other time, when I hold a
beloved book in my hand, my limitations fall
from me, my spirit is free.
Helen Keller from MIDSTREAM, 1930

THE YOUNAN FAMILY

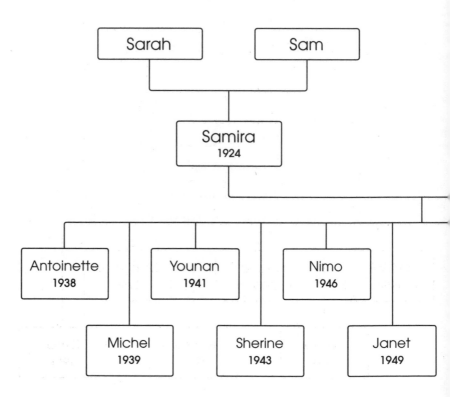

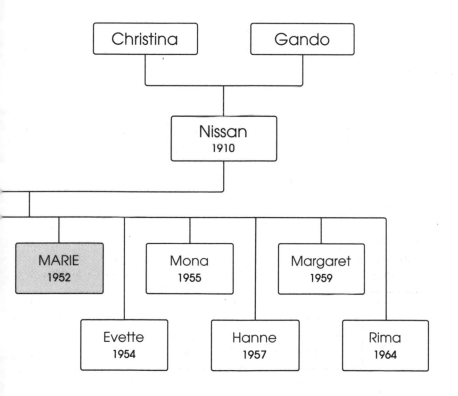

CONTENTS

Foreword

by Bill Jolley

deputy chair, Vision Australia

This is a compelling story of dispossession, frustration, hope, and triumph, beautifully written.

I knew Ben Hewitt, to whom Marie has dedicated her book. He was a kind and gentle man who mentored blind people by means as simple as his positive attitude, his serenity, his courtesy, and his patience. Marie became blinded when she was a baby, and had never been to school; it was Ben who brought her the gift of literacy through braille. Literacy unlocked Marie's capacity to learn English and to become qualified and employed as an interpreter.

I was born blind more than 60 years ago, but I was one of the lucky ones. My parents were loving, and held high expectations for me to get a good education and go on from there; Marie's parents were also loving, but they held no expectations for her to get an education, so there was nowhere for her to go on to. I was born and raised in sedate suburban Melbourne, not in a remote village in Syria.

I started learning braille in kindergarten and received a great education, which brought me friendships with other blind children and mentoring from adult role models; Marie sat at home with little to do but listen to her family, take in their stories, and eventually to teach herself Arabic.

I graduated from university in mathematics, and worked for many years until I retired by choice, whereas Marie was past 40 before she got her first pay cheque.

For all the above reasons, I am inspired by the stories of Marie's family and the Younan clan as they make their way in multicultural Australia — retaining the best of their rich Assyrian heritage whilst engaging with and contributing to our diverse mainstream community.

I have met blind people in Asia, Africa, and the Middle East as the Australian representative in the World Blind Union, and through my involvement in capacity-building aid projects. I have come to know that whilst many people in Australia who are blind or have low vision still struggle to achieve their goals, their counterparts in poorer countries face far greater challenges when disability, gender, poverty, civil unrest, and dislocation are compounded.

The 'siblinghood of blindness', I call it: those invisible bonds of friendship and empathy that transcend unimportant differences like colour, class, or creed. People who are blind the world over will empathise with Marie's challenges and triumphs as a blind person in a sighted world.

We can all recount times when we have had to shuffle forward into the darkness ahead, without a sighted guide or a cane to pave the way. We can all think of times when we haven't understood something, just because we couldn't see the obvious. And we can all revel in the mastering of new skills or the grasping of exciting opportunities that the kindness of a friend, or our own grit and determination, have unlocked.

As people who are blind or have low vision, we are fortunate in Australia to have access to rehabilitation and other services that compare favourably with world's best practice. Marie was taught braille and other independent living skills at the Royal Victorian Institute for the Blind, one of the three predecessor agencies that combined to form Vision Australia in 2004. One of our ongoing challenges at Vision Australia is to provide effective outreach to those migrant communities whose cultural norms may not include recognition of the capabilities and aspirations of blind people.

There is much in Marie's book for readers young and old to learn from, to enjoy, and upon which to reflect.

We can all reflect on the challenges faced by non-English-speaking migrants, recognise how lucky we are, and celebrate the outstanding contributions made by migrants to our commercial, civic, and cultural life.

And younger readers will enjoy a short, easy-to-read, true-life story about triumph over marginalisation and adversity. For here is the story of someone who grew up as an uneducated, disabled girl — assumed to be unemployable and unimportant — who became literate, knowledgeable, qualified, gainfully employed, and the much-loved matriarch of her extended family.

Thank you, Marie, for sharing your story. The retelling of your darkest nights and brightest days can teach us more than you will ever know.

Introduction

Thirty years ago, when I was a teacher at the Migrant Women's Learning Centre, a student with an engaging smile and a thirst for learning joined my class. Marie Younan was an Assyrian migrant who had been in Australia for twelve years. She had never been to school, was blind, and had recently acquired spoken English and basic literacy through learning braille at the Royal Victorian Institute for the Blind.

Marie joined a delightful group of migrant and refugee women who met for three days a week in the Return to Learning class. Here, they studied English language and literacy, while sharing their lives and fun in learning.

Whenever a new or unfamiliar word came up, I would write it on the whiteboard, while also saying each letter aloud so Marie could key it into her braille machine. With each new word she captured, her face would light up with joy.

One day, Marie told me how she had discovered as a child that she was blind. Her story stayed with me over the years and is written, almost word for word, as the first chapter in this book.

We kept in touch after we went our separate ways. Years later, at a MWLC reunion, Marie and I decided to work together to write the story of her life and educational journey.

When Marie started telling me the stories of her childhood, I was hooked. She is a mesmeric storyteller; I was drawn into her world as she told me about her years in Syria, Lebanon, Greece, and Melbourne. We agreed almost immediately that we would continue to work together to write her life history into a book, as Ben Hewitt had earlier encouraged her to do.

Over eight years, we met up in each other's homes. Marie told the stories of her life while I took notes, in awe of the details she had stored in her non-visual memory and the way she could create pictures in my mind of things she herself had never seen. I wrote her stories into chapters, which I would read to her at subsequent meetings. Each time Marie listened, she went more deeply into her previous life; new memories would come to the surface and she would relate new anecdotes, share new feelings, and discover new insights.

The book gradually took shape through many cycles of telling and writing, re-telling and re-writing.

Welcome to Marie's story!

Jill Sanguinetti

1
How Come You Can Get the Ball?

'How come you two can get the ball and I can't?'

Mona and Evette were throwing a ball to each other and putting it in my lap to throw back to them when they called my name. The ball had fallen on the floor, and I couldn't find it. I could never get the ball if it fell on the floor.

'Because you can't *see*. *We* can see, but you *can't*,' they said. 'That's why someone has to hold your hand and show you where everything is, because you're *blind*!'

I didn't understand at first. Then it dawned on me that there was a thing called 'seeing' that everyone else could do except me. Other people automatically knew where everything around them was, but I knocked into things and had to feel my way around the house.

I went over to where Mum was sitting and stood with my hands on the back of her cane chair.

'You look sad, Marie,' she said. 'What's wrong?'

'I just found out I'm different from my sisters, and you never told me.'

'That's alright,' she said. 'You're the same as all the others, only you can't see.'

I said nothing.

Mum's words still ring in my mind. I remember very little before that day. It was the day my life as a blind person began.

What did it mean, to see, or not to see? At the tender age of seven, I thought about it all the time and began to realise how different I really was.

2
A Little Family History

I was born in a village called Tel Wardiyat, in the top right-hand corner of Syria that pokes between Turkey to the north and Iraq to the east. It's on flat farming land along the Khabur River, a tributary of the Euphrates; cold in winter and baking hot in summer.

I'm *Assyrian*, not Syrian, even though I was born in Syria. Assyrians descend from the ancient kingdom of Assyria that ruled over Mesopotamia more than 2,000 years ago. We are Christians and we speak Aramaic, the closest living language to the language Jesus would have spoken. Being blind, I've never seen Assyrian writing, but I'm told it looks like Hebrew, with 22 letters going from right to left.

Before I tell you the rest of my story, I need to tell you a little about my family history and my grandparents' stories of survival and escape a hundred years ago.

•

For centuries, Christian communities living in the Ottoman Empire suffered discrimination and oppression as infidels. Between 1894 and 1924, more than three million Armenian, Greek, and Assyrian Christians were killed by the Ottomans, another two million were expelled, and thousands of women were raped and forcibly converted to Islam.

The killing of millions of Christians by Turks, Kurds, and Arabs in the early part of the twentieth century is now recognised by many nations as genocide. We Assyrians call that terrible part of our history the *Sayfo*, or Sword.

My four grandparents, Sarah, Sam, Christina, and Gando, were refugees several times over during the years of the *Sayfo*.

They all came from a mountainous region in southern Turkey called Hakkari, which for centuries was a homeland of Assyrian tribes. In 1914, they were driven from their homes by the Ottoman army along with thousands of other Assyrians and forced to walk to neighbouring Iran. They survived hunger, exposure, and mass killings on the 100-kilometre march. Many more were killed in Iran as they tried to get to the city of Urmia, where there was a large Assyrian community that also came under attack.

They later escaped from Urmia, and for the next 12 years, they lived as refugees, moving between different countries as they tried to eke out a living.

Sarah, Sam, Christina, and Gando often travelled together during those years of migration and displacement. Many of their children and other relatives were killed or died along the way.

My father, Nissan, was born in Hakkari in 1910. His parents, Gando and Christina, were expelled from their home village when he was four years old. Gando and Christina became separated when they were walking with thousands of other Assyrians to northern Iran. Eventually they met up again and made their way safely to Russia.

Dad was the only one of Gando and Christina's four children to survive the 12 years they spent travelling from place to place as refugees. They lived in Moscow for four years, then migrated to Greece where they lived for another eight years, so Dad grew up speaking Russian and Greek, as well as Assyrian, Turkish, and Arabic. Dad was 16 in 1926 when the British Mandate was governing Mesopotamia and the family moved from Greece to Iraq under British protection.

They went to a village called Duhok in Kurdistan, near

Mosul, where they lived for eight years while Dad and Gando worked as agricultural labourers.

The British were supporting the formation of an independent Iraqi army so that they could withdraw their forces when Iraq became an independent country. At the same time, they needed to defend British army bases against Arab and Kurdish rebellions. Assyrian soldiers were prized by the British for their fierce fighting skills and their Christian religion, so they were recruited to serve in the British army during the period of transition. But when the British pulled out in 1933, Arabs and Kurds took revenge on the Assyrians. Up to 3,000 were killed by gangs in what became known as the Simele massacre. In 1934, when Dad was about 24, the family once again fled from great danger, this time to the village of Tel Wardiyat, across the Syrian border in the Hasakah province.

At that time, Syria was governed by the French Mandate. Like the British, the French favoured the Assyrians because, as the Assyrians were a Christian minority in a Muslim country, the French expected loyalty from them. With the support of the League of Nations, the French gave land to about 6,000 Assyrians who had been driven out by the Simele massacre, and more followed over the next decade. Tel Wardiyat was one of 30 villages established for the Assyrians along the Khabur

River in the Hasakah region in north-eastern Syria.

A few years after Dad arrived in Tel Wardiyat with his parents, his father died. As the only child, Dad was responsible for his mother and cared for her for the rest of her long life.

Mum's parents, Sarah and Sam, fled to Russia with Christina and Gando then moved to Iraq in 1919. There they lived in a village near Mosul called Zakho, where Mum — Samira — was born in 1924. Sarah and Sam had 18 babies all together, but only six of them survived into adulthood.

In 1926, when Mum was about two, Sam was recruited into the Assyrian Levies along with several thousand Assyrians, Kurds, Armenians, and Marsh Arabs. In 1927, he was sent with his family to Hamidiya, near Baghdad, where the Assyrian Levies were guarding the Royal Air Force base. He was given a house, a salary, and weekly rations. The British built an Assyrian school where Mum and her brothers and sisters had a few years of primary schooling. That is where Mum learned to read Assyrian and to recite some prayers in English. Grandfather Sam told me that the Assyrians would sometimes go out to hunt deer when they were not on duty. They would eat the meat, and give the heads to the British officers, to be stuffed and mounted on a wall.

Sam served in the Assyrian Levies from 1926 to 1933, when the Simele massacre broke out and Sam and his family were evacuated. Mum was nine when they left Hamidiya and travelled by military camion to Tel Wardiyat. When Dad, Gando, and Christina arrived a year later, the two families were once again reunited.

Dad saw Mum for the first time in 1934, when she was collecting sticks with a group of young girls at a family wedding party in Tel Wardiyat. He thought she was beautiful with her fair hair and blue eyes, and made up his mind to marry her, even though she was only ten, and, at 24, he was more than twice her age. Christina asked Sam and Sarah for Mum's hand in marriage before the two young people had met or spoken with each other. Both families were delighted about the match. They had already hoped that their children would one day marry to seal the family friendship.

Mum and Dad married in 1937, when she was 13 — even before she had her first period. She often told us the story of her childhood marriage. At first, she thought Dad's proposal was a joke and refused him outright. Why would she want to marry a grown man she didn't even know? She told me that her aunt came to the door one day with a pair of new shoes for her to wear at her wedding. Mum locked the door and yelled, 'I'm not opening the door for you! I'm not getting married! *You c*an put on the shoes and get married!'

Mum eventually accepted that she really had no choice — in those days, young girls had little say in the matter. Her mother told her that Christina would be like a second mother and would care for her like her own daughter.

After they married, Mum went to live with Dad, Christina, and Gando, and helped with the housework and farm work. She grew to love her husband and especially loved her mother-in-law, who became our grandmother or 'Yima'. Yima was head of our family and lived with us until she died in Melbourne in 1978, at the age of 100.

Mum had her first child, Antoinette, in 1938, when she was just 14. She didn't know about the facts of life before getting pregnant for the first time, and, after that, she was pregnant most of the time, which meant she hardly ever had a period. Antoinette was quickly followed by two boys, Michel and Younan. Then came nine more girls: Sherine, Nimo, Janet, Marie (me), Evette, Mona, Hanne, Margaret, and Rima. Another boy died when he was a few weeks old, so Mum had 13 babies altogether.

I was born in 1952, right in the middle. By the time I was five or six, Antoinette had married and moved to her own home in another village so I didn't get to know her very well until years later. Antoinette and Sherine were pregnant with their oldest children at the same time as Mum was pregnant with her younger ones, so my three youngest sisters, Hanne, Margaret, and Rima, have nieces and nephews who are all the same age as they are.

The old people didn't talk much about the *Sayfo* or their refugee experiences. Dad must have remembered his refugee years, as he was 16 when they finally returned from Russia and went to live in the Assyrian community in Iraq. But he never talked about the suffering; he just told us funny stories about when he was an apprentice shoemaker in Greece. Grandfather Sam never talked about his traumatic experiences either. He only told us stories about life in the army camp and how good the British were. But on wet winter afternoons, Yima's and Sarah's friends would come to sit around the fire and chat. The old ladies would tell stories that began, 'Do you remember such and such …?' I was the only one who was hearing the grandmothers' stories — my brothers and sisters would be off doing other things.

That is how I heard what happened to them in 1914,

when they were forced to take their children and leave their homes in Hakkari to walk to Iran with little or no food or shelter.

It was on a Sunday, and Sarah had a casserole of *dolma* (stuffed vine leaves) boiling on the fire. They had planned an early lunch because they thought something bad might happen. Suddenly, they received an order to leave the house and start walking, and the lunch was left uneaten. Sarah told us how much she longed for the *dolma* when they were walking for days in the bitter cold with almost nothing to eat.

At around the same time, Yima was also forced onto the road, carrying Dad, aged four or five, and a bag of belongings. Separated from her husband, she became so exhausted that she had to keep putting Dad and her bag on the ground and resting before she could keep going.

Most people had large families, and parents could not carry all their children or feed them, so they would leave their children along the road, promising to come back soon to collect them. They knew they would not come back, but they hoped that others coming along behind them might pick them up. One day, Yima saw her little cousin Joanna abandoned on the roadside, so she took her by the hand and rescued her. Joanna survived and later lived near us in Tel Wardiyat.

The Ottomans were killing Assyrian men and forcing thousands of others, mainly women and children, to walk across the border into Iran. One day, the women were herded into a building surrounded by a high wall. Yima crept out of the building and looked out through a crack in the high wall. She saw hundreds of bodies piled up beyond the wall. She knew her sister, brother-in-law, and their four children had all been killed, so she tried to see if their bodies were there, but when she saw all the bodies, she fainted.

Miriam, another one of Yima's cousins, was locked up in the building with them. Miriam screamed when she saw the bodies of her uncle, her father, and brother. A soldier hit her with the butt of his gun, took her out, and told her to step onto the bodies of her family. In the end, she stepped on her father and her uncle, but she refused to step on her brother. After that, they continued walking to Iran.

Another time, a group of women and children were locked up together. They killed one woman's son, and she lost her mind. She took all her clothes off and started running around attacking all the other women with a stick. The soldiers told them to push the mad woman towards the door. When they did, they took her out and shot her.

Yima kept Joanna with her while they were walking through Iran to get to Russia. Joanna was wearing a brightly coloured silk scarf. One day, a soldier came up to her, ripped the scarf from her head, and pulled her hair. Many, many years later, when I went to Chicago in 1995, I met Joanna who was by then very old, in her late 80s. I asked her if she remembered the Iranian soldier ripping off her scarf. She said she could remember crying when the soldier stole her scarf. Yima had said to her, 'Don't worry, I'll buy you another one.'

Yima and Gando were reunited and continued travelling to Russia by foot and horse-drawn cart, arriving in 1916. Russia was a Christian country and an enemy of the Ottoman Empire, so Assyrians thought they would be safe there. They arrived at the start of the Russian revolution. They didn't dare take sides. If anyone knocked on the door, they would pretend they were on the side of that person.

Yima and Gando lived in Russia for five years, then in Greece for eight years, before moving to Iraq. During those years, Yima had three more babies, two boys and a girl, but two died in Russia and the third in Greece.

I don't remember Sarah talking about the babies she lost when they were travelling as refugees. She did tell us about the time when they were walking with no fresh water to drink. Everyone had to drink from a filthy yellow roadside puddle. Afterwards some people got sick and died. She also told us that when the soles of her shoes were worn out, she had to keep on walking, even though her feet were cut and bleeding. She said that more than 30 years later, she could still feel the pain in her feet from those days.

3
Tel Wardiyat: Hill of Flowers

Tel Wardiyat means 'hill of flowers'. I remember the flowers. With my tiny bit of sight, I could just make out patches of yellow and white where flowers were growing along the roadside.

We were a family of 15: parents, Samira and Nissan; grandmother Christina; and 12 children. We spoke Assyrian at home and strictly observed our Assyrian Christian religion while living peacefully alongside our Muslim neighbours.

Yima was our matriarch — proud, loving, and hardworking. She was born in 1878, so she was 74 when I was born. She made all the main decisions and did the farm work, food preparation, and cooking.

Dad was responsible for earning an income, but

accepted his mother's authority over the running of the household and family matters.

Mum was second in command after Yima, in charge of washing, cleaning, child-minding, and clothes-making. She sewed, knitted, or crocheted our clothes, made pillows and doonas out of feathers plucked from our hens and ducks, and sewed mattresses filled with wool that Yima sheared from our single sheep.

Mum and Yima got on well and worked as a team to look after us. But Yima's word was law. She didn't let Mum cut our hair, so every morning we girls lined up for her to braid our long hair, one by one. She never complained about her problems or the fact that three of her four children, and many relatives, had died in the *Sayfo*.

We called Mum 'Yimi', which is Assyrian for mother. She could read and write in Assyrian a little bit, thanks to her few years' schooling in the British school at Hamadiya. She would read to us from the Bible and say, 'Jesus said, "love your God, then love your neighbour, then love yourself". You should give to poor people, help poor people: if anyone comes to the house to ask for anything, just give it to them; if anyone asks you for help, just help them.' We were neither rich nor poor, but we had enough for ourselves and always gave to people in need. Yima couldn't read or write, having never been to school, but she too would tell us that we should be like Jesus and be kind to other people.

Dad, our 'Baba', was a mechanic in charge of the machinery on a big cotton and wheat farm, and was away from home much of the time. He was easy-going and loved all his kids, especially me. He would watch out for me more than the others and call me to have a coffee with him. When he came home after a few days away at work, he would be laden with food and gifts. He would empty his pockets of change, hand out coins, and tell stories and jokes. He was very outgoing, and would always welcome friends and new acquaintances to our home. Like his mother, he became known and loved in the community for helping people in different ways.

Mum's parents, Sarah and Sam, were also called 'Yima' and 'Baba'. They lived next door with their two unmarried sons (my uncles) and spent most of their time with us, so our house was usually full of people. Sam spoke a little English and was like a British gentleman — very fussy about his house, his dress, and food. Everything in his garden had to be perfect — even the trees had to be pruned to the same size. If I came inside with muddy shoes, he would tease me, saying he would give lollies to all the other girls, except me, because I was naughty. I would answer him back cheekily, saying 'I don't care, I don't want any lollies.'

Sarah, my other Yima, was a quiet lady who always kept in the background. Like Christina, she had never learned to read or write. She always seemed sad and never said very much. I knew it was because she had lost so many children and family members when they were refugees. Sometimes I would hear her crying or quietly praying, and I felt sorry for all the tragedies in her life.

Sam, Sarah, and their two sons went to live in Beirut in 1963, when I was 11. Sam died shortly after, and I didn't meet Sarah again until four years later, when we went to Lebanon.

In the early days, it was like having five parents who all took part in looking after us — our Mum and Dad (Samira and Nissan); Mum's parents (Sarah and Sam); and Yima (Christina). I loved Yima the most, because she was at the centre of the household and made me her favourite.

I couldn't see shapes or people, but I knew if it was day or night, and I could make out colours: the blue of the sky, the red of sunsets, the green of trees, and the yellow of flowers. I loved those colours and remember them to this day, even though I became totally blind more than 30 years ago.

I developed my own special walk — sliding my feet forward on the ground while leaning my body back, so if there were any obstacles, my feet would bump into them first. When we went out, I had to take someone's arm and I would walk with my head back, looking up, because the sky was all I could see. Mum used to say, 'Don't walk like that with your head back; you look funny.'

Life on our small plot of land at Tel Wardiyat was peaceful and secure. We had a paddock with two cows, a donkey, a sheep, ducks, hens, and turkeys. Dad rented a few acres of land just outside the village, where he grew vegetables and a crop of cotton every year. All my brothers and sisters helped pick the cotton and pile it into sacks to be taken away on the donkey's back. Dad also grew wheat on a plot of land further away in the hills. Every year, he harvested the wheat and ground it into flour in the electricity-driven mill shared by the villagers of Tel Wardiyat.

Yima produced eggs, vegetables, and fruit, and milk that she made into cheese and butter. She made jams and pickles, and crushed grapes to make wine that she kept in a small outside shed. She would kill and pluck chooks for us to eat and buy meat from neighbours whenever they killed a lamb or calf. Sometimes she would buy fruit and vegetables from a man who went past every day, selling all sorts of things from his donkey cart.

I remember the sounds and smells of Tel Wardiyat: the summer smell of dry grass in the yard and laneways; the high, squealing voices of children playing; the hens clucking, the cows mooing, and the dog barking. I loved listening to the wind swishing through the trees and smelling their fresh smell. I especially remember the crackling sound of Yima's cooking fire, which burned constantly and kept the family warm in winter, and the welcoming smell of the pumpkin, sunflower, and sesame seeds she toasted on the iron hotplate. Every day, the house was filled with the delicious smell of Yima's soups and stews and Mum's fresh flatbread.

The backyard smelled of cows, chooks, and our hole-in-the-ground toilet. I learned to go up to the cows on my own, stroke them, and put my face right up against their hides so I could see their black and white markings. Once, Yima got me to hold a cow's udder and try to milk it, but there was something yucky about the feel of the smooth, rubbery teats and the warm milk coming out.

Our house was made of mud brick, white-washed on the inside. I could just make out the single blue stripe that was painted around the middle of each wall. We had a big family room in which we all lived and the children played, and a special sitting room reserved for visitors. There were four bedrooms — one for Mum and Dad and the youngest babies, one for the two boys, another for the girls, and a small room that Yima shared with my younger sister Evette. Mattresses were stacked against the wall during the day and laid on the floor at night. There was no electricity, just kerosene lamps for light, and a fire for cooking and warming the main room.

Every day, the girls went to the cement-lined canal a few hundred metres away to get buckets of water for washing ourselves and our clothes. The boys never carried the water — only the girls. Sometimes I was allowed to help by carrying a bucket in each hand after someone had filled it. Carrying the water was about the only thing I could do that made me feel useful.

The water was then boiled in a large metal container made from half a petrol drum. The other half of the drum was used to store drinking water in the kitchen. On bath days, you had to mix hot and cold water in another container and sit on a wooden bench to wash yourself. If you were the last person to use all the warm water, you had to fill the container with warm water for the next person. The water was warmed by burning dried cotton plants, left over from the cotton harvest, and sticks gathered from trees that grew along the Khabur River.

Drinking water had to be brought from the river. The girls would walk down with the donkey, fill four 20-litre tin containers, load them in baskets on each side of the donkey, and lead him back. Later, my brother Younan made a wooden trolley lined with metal, so we could bring back water from the river more easily. The trolley carried twice as much water as the donkey did, but it was too heavy for the girls to pull. Because of that, Younan had to help them drag it back home, even though getting water was supposed to be girls' work.

We all used the same pit toilet, which went straight into the ground. I kept a small stick in the toilet for feeling where the hole was, so I knew where to put my feet when I squatted. To get to the toilet, I had to brave the hens. Somehow, they knew I couldn't see them or defend myself, so they bullied me by running after me and pecking the backs of my legs. They never pecked any of the other children, just me. My legs would be covered with little lumps where they had pecked me, so sometimes I stayed inside as long as I could to avoid the chook attacks.

I was also terrified of the dog and cat, because Yima said they might bite or scratch me. Our dog must have known I was blind, because he would give a special little growl when he saw me coming, to warn me not to tread on him.

Moths were my worst horror. We didn't have flywire screens on the windows, so every night, moths and other insects would fly into the house. Whenever I felt them fluttering against my hair or face, I would scream hysterically. I never saw the moths, but knew they were my enemy, like secret attackers from another world.

Every now and then, I would sneak out of the house to have a little walk on my own in nearby laneways, although I wasn't supposed to do this. Sometimes I would lose my way, and I'd have to stop and go over in my mind where I had been and where everything was around me before I could find my way again.

One day, when no-one was watching, I took two buckets and found my way down to the canal. I could just see the green line where grass grew next to the dirt track, so I followed it down to the water. In order to fill the buckets, I had to feel for the chain that I knew was attached to a ladder in the water, then hold onto it. I filled the buckets and brought them home without telling anyone. Yima saw me, though, and threatened to tell my brothers what I had done. Being boys, they were supposed to discipline us girls. Nothing happened, but I felt proud that when we were running short of water, I had dared do something on my own to help. I learned I *could* do things on my own if I really wanted to.

Yima was strict but loving. She taught us to share everything and never allowed us to fight. We children were well-behaved, and we played together all day in the house and yard. There were never any arguments or tensions. When we had visitors, we had to stay in the children's room. If we ran around the house and made a noise, Yima would say, 'Shame on you, you didn't respect yourself or other people, and you didn't respect me.' Then she would give us a pretend smack, like a pat, and say, 'I'm just giving your clothes a little brush.' She never hit us, because she believed it would make us stubborn, and because she loved us too much. I remember Mum's friend once asking, 'Why are you brushing their clothes — they are quite clean?'

With so many sisters, we had to do everything together. All the girls' clothes were kept together in a big wooden box, so if anyone wanted anything, they had to sort through it. Mum would buy the material for our dresses from a man who went from door to door with big rolls of cloth on his back, and we were allowed to choose our own colours. We got new clothes every Christmas and Easter, when everything had to be new. Later, the new clothes went into the common clothes box to be shared. My clothes were in a separate box to make it easier for me to find them. All the clothes were washed by hand and dried on a line in the yard. Our best dresses were hung along one wall after Mum ironed them with the flat iron. She would catch the bus to Hasakah to buy shoes and other clothes in bulk. In winter, we wore flat shoes with thin, bendy soles and a little ribbon on top, and we wore sandals in summer.

We grew our fruit and vegetables on a nearby plot of land that Dad rented. Yima did most of the gardening, collected the vegies, planned the meals, and did all the cooking. For breakfast we had bread, cheese, eggs, olives, jam, and tea or milk. Our main meal was in the middle of the day; mainly soups or stews, which we ate with rice and Mum's flatbread. Yima would put the hot casserole and a large platter containing all the other food on the floor. We'd sit cross-legged in a circle while she gave us a bowl, called our names, and served us one by one. We were not allowed to touch the casserole and had to eat everything we were given. If we cleaned our plate properly, we could have more. After we had turned 15, we could have a glass of her home-made wine with our meal. In the evening, we would have bread and leftovers from lunch with fruit, warm milk, cocoa, or tea made from wild camomile flowers that grew along the road.

Yima had a rule that we were never allowed to say we were hungry. She would say, 'I've seen people fainting from hunger and dying from hunger. Don't say "I'm hungry," because you are not really hungry. Just say, "I'd like something to eat."'

Every Easter and Christmas we had to fast, which meant no meat, chicken, or dairy foods for 50 days before Easter (Lent) or 25 days before Christmas (Advent). Instead we ate fruit and salads, vegetables cooked in oil, or bread dipped in tahini. Relatives and friends would come to eat with us during fasting times. People used to say that our house was important, because so many visitors would come to eat with us during Lent and Advent.

Every Easter, Yima would make hard-boiled Easter eggs and dye them red with cochineal, which is called *kirmiz in* Assyrian. She would also use *kirmiz to* make pink cakes, and to dye our bed-socks red. Sometimes the children pretended to be monsters by putting *kirmiz* into their eyes to make their eyeballs go red. Yima told us that the *kirmiz* was expensive, as it was made out of the crushed bodies of small insects that lived under the ground in Turkey.

All my brothers and sisters went to school except me. Everyone thought school would be wasted on me because, being blind, I would not be able to read or learn anything. When the others went to school in the morning, I had to stay home with the toddlers and babies. When they came home from school and did their homework, I would sit and hold their schoolbooks, wondering what was in them. I wished I could read and write like them. That was my one big wish. But I said to myself, 'I will never be able to read or write because I'm blind.'

When the others went out to weddings and parties, I had to stay home with Yima. Sometimes I cried when I found myself alone, and she would say, 'I've got some lollies here, I'll give you a lolly.' Sometimes the house just went quiet, and I realised they had all slipped out without telling me, including Yima.

Sometimes I tried to join in their game of hide and seek by feeling for hiding places and listening for my sisters' footsteps and giggles, but no matter how hard I tried, I always got left out.

Assyrian children celebrate Halloween by dressing up and going to the neighbours' houses early in the morning for 'trick or treat', and I always wished I could go with them. One year they took me, but I missed out on the fun because I couldn't see the costumes or the people who came to the doors. After that I decided not to go again, because it would only make me sad.

Mum had all her babies at home. I loved it when the babies came, because the whole family would be excited and joyful. I was too scared to hold them when they were tiny, in case I dropped them. When they were older, I would sometimes be given a baby to cuddle, but I always gave her back after a few minutes. It was a sad thing to hold a baby and not be able to look into her face, to see her smile, or see who she looked like, or what her eyes were telling me. My sisters could make the babies laugh and smile. I could talk to them, but I had no real way of communicating with them.

I spent a lot of time thinking about my blindness and all the things my sisters could do that I couldn't or wasn't allowed to do. They lived in light while I lived in thick fog. The colours that shone faintly through the fog reminded me of what they had, but I did not. By the time I was eight or nine, I began to withdraw from my sisters. I would listen to them playing, but not try to join in because I couldn't really play with them. I knew I was locked out of their world. It was better to live inside my own little world and my own mind than try to be in their world and fail.

The highlight of my week was when we all went to church on Sunday mornings. I liked the walk through the village, the sound of the priest singing and chanting prayers, and the sacred smell of incense. Church was a holy place where I was loved equally as one of God's children. We learned about Jesus and the Holy Father, how to be good Christians, and how to live well so we would go to heaven in the next life. On Easter Sunday, we would hold candles during the service. I loved seeing the bright circles of light, and would stare into my own flickering candle for as long as I could before I put it out, afraid that I would accidentally knock into someone and burn them.

Every Christmas and Easter, the priest came to bless our house. We had to line up to kiss his hand and then kiss the cross after he put it on our heads. We had to behave ourselves when he was there, and we weren't allowed in the room while he was eating.

My sisters were always chattering and laughing, but as the blind one I was an outsider, listening more than taking part. Nimo, three years older than me, was the sister who looked after me the most. She would take me by the hand and try to include me when she could. Because I was dependent on them for so much, I learned early to contain my feelings and not be demanding. I had to make up for being blind by being extra good.

I had one girlfriend, a relative on my father's side called Yola, who was the same age as me and lived across the road from our house. Yola would hold my hand and talk about everything and bring me lollies, grapes, or apricots. She would often invite me to her home. There wasn't much traffic in those days, so I could find my way on my own. She would make sandwiches and tea for me, and we would sit together and talk. Then we would go for a walk while she described everything that was around us. She told me the names and colours of the different flowers and got me to smell them. Yola was the one who taught me how to braid my hair on my own. Now she lives in London with her family. She is still my friend, and every now and then we talk on the phone.

Of all the cousins and relatives who would come to visit — so many that I could never learn their names or remember them all — there was one family I loved more than the others: Mum's youngest sister, Yonia, her husband, Samuel, and their children. When they came to visit, they would always make me laugh. Samuel was a doctor in a nearby village. His first wife had died, and he was much older than Yonia, but his spirit was young, and he loved telling jokes.

When I was about ten, Mum and Dad took me to a doctor, who said I might get my sight back if I had a corneal transplant. But Yima and Dad said, 'How could they do that? No-one can transplant a cornea, it is not possible.' So they didn't give me the operation.

Then, when I was about 12, a relative said to Mum, 'If you want, I'll take Marie to a boarding school for blind girls and bring her home every fortnight.' Mum wanted me to go. She said I might learn something and grow up with knowledge. But Yima said I couldn't go; that I wouldn't be able to learn anything because I couldn't see. She said, 'If she goes far away from us something might happen to her, maybe she will die.' Dad said, 'I've got 12 children, and I'm not sending one to boarding school, especially if she's disabled.' I was heartbroken. Why wouldn't they let me go? I said to Mum, 'I don't know anything about the world, or about life. Why can't I live, and take a risk? I wish I was dead. Isn't it better to take a risk and be happy?'

When I was 13, I got a tummy ache and my pants felt wet. No-one had told me anything about periods, so I changed my pants, but I didn't know what was happening. My sisters saw me and said, 'You're in trouble!' Then they told Yima, and she explained that all females bleed once a month, and I would have to wear a pad when it happened. Being blind, it was hard to know when I had a period, but I learned to hold the toilet paper up to my eyes to see if there was a little bit of red. When I saw the blood, it was alright because I knew. After that, Yima kept a special bag for my pads and looked after me when I got my period.

The pads were made out of old rags. The other girls had to wash theirs and hang them on the line, but I didn't have to.

Nobody thought to read to me or find things for me to do. Not that they were cruel; they were busy with their own lives, though, and didn't take much notice of me. I was just there. I didn't have any toys or games of my own, apart from a rag doll Mum made for me with little arms and legs, and buttons sewed on for eyes. But the doll scared me — there was something creepy about it.

So, for most of the time, there was nothing to occupy me at home. I would sit on a chair in my corner and do nothing — just play with my fingers or run my hand around the hem of my skirt for hours on end. I listened to the conversations going on around me, and every day passed the same as the one before. Because I didn't go to school, I wasn't sent to bed at 9pm like the others and could stay up with the adults for as long as I liked. During the day and in the evenings, I listened to their conversations, family stories, and anecdotes, and took in their wisdom. My mind was the book in which I wrote down everything that happened in the family.

One day, when I was quietly listening, they were talking about how sad it was that I was blind. Yima said to Mum,

'I will never forgive myself for making her go blind. Why did I put that *kirmiz* in her eyes?'

I said nothing, but my mind was in turmoil. Could it have been Yima, whom I loved more than anyone else in the world, who had made me go blind? Did she really blind me by putting *kirmiz* (cochineal) in my eyes? Why did no-one ever talk to me about my blindness, or teach me how to do things? I was full of questions, but didn't dare ask, and I never talked about it with anyone in the family. I thought over and over about how guilty Yima must have felt about blinding me by accident.

My life changed for the better when I was about 14, and they bought me a small transistor radio. At last I had something to do. I would listen all day, every day, in my corner, gradually teaching myself to understand Arabic. Before that, I only spoke and understood Assyrian, although I heard Arabic spoken when vendors came up and down the street with their donkey carts.

I got to know the popular Arabic songs and tried to piece together what the words meant. If I heard words I didn't know, I would memorise them and ask my sisters what they meant when they came home from school. With no responsibilities and little stimulation, my mind was empty, so I was ready and eager to absorb new information from the radio. The others could speak Arabic because they went to an Arabic school in the village. I would sit with them at the table while they were doing their homework. I listened to them reading aloud, and asked them to say in Assyrian what the words meant, training myself to memorise instead of writing things down. Once they told me the meaning of an Arabic word, I never forgot it. Listening to the radio and learning Arabic from my sisters gave me an inkling of what life beyond our home and village might be like.

I craved Mum's attention and would sometimes try to grab her dress when she walked by. But she had to share her attention with so many people: her husband, her mother-in-law, her mother, father, and her 12 children. She was always kind and supportive, and I knew she was there for me, even though she had so many others to care for. I felt closest to her on the rare occasions she took me out to go to the doctor or go shopping. They were the only times I had her to myself.

Yima was a tower of strength and generosity. My brother-in-law Peter once said, 'On every finger she has a candle.' This was because her hands were always open and giving to everyone. If homeless people came by, or people were caught in the rain, she always sheltered them or gave things to them. She was an important person in the village — everyone called her 'auntie', and even the mayor of the village used to call to ask her advice. Yima was warm and charismatic, a natural leader who needed to be in control. Dad couldn't make any decisions about the family without her consent. Even when young men came to ask if they could marry one of my sisters, it was Yima, not Mum or Dad, who made the decision.

I was her favourite, but she over-protected me. She was like a security guard, watching me in case I fell or hurt myself, and making sure I didn't go with the rest of the family to weddings and parties. I only remember going to one party, at which I heard someone say, 'Why is she here? She's blind!' Mum said, 'Yes, but she can hear, and if she hears something happy, it will make her happy. Her heart is alive.' Mum understood, but with Yima in charge, she couldn't do much to get me out of the house or make my life more interesting. As a result, I became more and more insecure and dependent on them both.

Christmas, Easter, weddings, church outings, and family comings and goings went on around me, but my real life went on inside my head. I thought about things and took a mental note of everything that happened.

Learning Arabic kept my mind alive and gave me a purpose. My sisters were my constant companions, but Yola was the one who gave me friendship and a life outside the family, at least until she moved to Beirut when I was 14.

I knew I would always have to live at home with them because, as they so often said, 'Blind girls don't get married.' They didn't know that I could learn to do many things, or that disabled people have needs and rights the same as everyone else. They did the best they could, given the times and the attitudes of the day.

But for all their love and care, I was locked in an empty world, like being in a cage with a blanket thrown over the top.

4
Beirut:
Escape from Civil War

Life in Tel Wardiyat stayed the same until 1967, the year I turned 15. Yima was 89, and could no longer keep up with the milking, the cheese-making, gardening, food preparation, and cooking. Mum could not take on Yima's work *and* look after the large family still at home.

By then, my oldest sisters Antoinette, Sherine, and Nimo had married and left home. Sherine and Nimo were living in Beirut with their families. Grandmother Sarah had also moved to Beirut with her sons and their families. So Mum, Dad, and Yima decided that we too would go to Beirut, where we could live more comfortably, join the rest of the family, and buy food from shops. There would be more opportunities for my brothers and sisters to find work. As well, Beirut would be safe because it had a Christian government. I was overjoyed at the prospect, because Yola and her family had been living in Beirut for a year by then. Life in a big city would be more exciting, I said to myself, than being stuck at home all day in a tiny village.

Dad had to work out how to move the family to Beirut, 800 kilometres away, find a job, and set up a new home there. It was a complicated operation, so he moved us in two stages. Mum went first with Younan (25), me (15), Mona (13), Evette (12), and four-year-old Rima. Dad stayed on in Tel Wardiyat for another six months, with Yima, Michel (26), Janet (14), Margaret (7), and nine-year-old Hanne.

Early one April morning in 1967, six of us, Mum and the five children, climbed into the bus to Hasakah with our bags and suitcases. There, we boarded another bus that took us on the ten-hour trip through Homs and Aleppo to Damascus. The bus bumped and lurched, the engine roared, and brakes screeched as we listened to pop songs on the crackly radio and breathed in petrol fumes and dust. At last we arrived in Damascus and hopped onto another bus that took us for two hours across the border to Beirut.

Dad had rented an apartment for us in Haddad, a suburb near the centre of the city in the Christian quarter, close to other Assyrian families. It was smaller than our house in the village but more comfortable. For the first time, we had a proper inside toilet, electricity, hot running water, and a shower. We girls would line up and run in and out after each other to wash while the shower was left running.

Six months later, Dad packed up the house and drove the rest of the family in a truck to Beirut: Yima and the two little ones in the front, and Michel and Janet in the back with all our belongings. He found a job in a factory that made plastic shoes, plates, and containers. We were happy to be together again and settled quickly into city life.

We were in the same apartment block where Sarah and my uncles' families lived — we were on the first floor and they were on the second floor. I was allowed to go up and down the stairs to visit them whenever I wanted to. I could also walk to visit Dad's cousins, who lived a few houses down, by feeling the buildings and doors along the way. The family visits gave me a little bit of independence. But most of the time I had to stay inside, even when the others were going out to dinners and parties.

Life was easier for Mum and Yima now that we could buy our food instead of feeding ourselves from our small farm and garden. Yima had slowed down but still did much of the cooking and housework, and kept a watchful eye over everything I did. Her questioning and supervision became harder to bear: 'What are you drinking?' 'What are you eating?' 'What is in your hand?' I was suffocating under her constant monitoring and control, but I respected her too much to resist.

Physically I was an adult, but emotionally still a child, because I had no way of growing up in the outside world. Nobody had told me the facts of life or the difference between men's and women's bodies, so I didn't understand why girls all slept in one room and boys in another, or why people had to go into a room and shut the door behind them when they changed their clothes. By 16, I was longing to be able to meet new people and learn about how they lived in the outside world. More than anything, I wanted a life of my own that I could have more control over.

My older brothers and sisters were married or marrying, and dispersing to other parts of the world. Antoinette's husband, Peter, had gone to Melbourne by ship in 1966, followed in 1967 by Antoinette and their four children. Our eldest brother, Michel, married in 1969, migrated to Melbourne with his wife, Rosa, and their two daughters, and found a good job in the Ford car factory in Campbellfield. Sisters

Nimo and Mona migrated to America with their husbands and children, and Sherine had gone to live in Beirut in 1960, after she was married there.

Then Yima decided to go to Melbourne to be with Michel and his family. She was still quite sprightly and flew there with Janet and Evette. Mum cried when she left, as they were very close. Dad was pleased, thinking that soon we would all be reunited in Australia. I knew I would miss Yima, but I was secretly happy to be free of her control.

My greatest joy was when Yola came to visit or take me out. She had joined a Protestant Assyrian church run by an American minister called 'Brother Hans', who spoke Arabic. One day, Yola took me to church with her and introduced me to her friends there. I was quite fluent in Arabic by then and could understand everything. After a while, Brother Hans asked if I would like to become a member of the church. I said he would have to ask Mum and Dad for permission. I knew Yima would not have allowed it, but now she was in Australia, they were free to decide for themselves. Dad could make his own decisions for the first time, even though by then he was in his 50s. Brother Hans came to our home, told Mum and Dad about the church, and gave Dad a Bible. They agreed to let me join. At last I had a social life in Beirut, outside of the family, and people my own age to get to know.

I was 19 when they let me go on a church camp in the hills amongst the cedar trees. We went for walks, played games, had barbeques, and studied the Bible sitting under the trees. Eight-year-old Rima was there as my guide and chaperone. I made new friends, laughed with them, and felt as if I was coming alive at last. But soon I was home again, with few chances to get out of the house or go anywhere on my own, apart from church.

One day, I plucked up courage to ask Mum how I became blind, and what Yima had done. Mum told me that when I was six months old, I had contracted an eye infection. At that time, there was an American doctor travelling around villages in our area and helping people with eye problems. A friend of the family told Mum she should take me to him. He prescribed eye drops, and told Mum he would come back in a month to check on me. Sadly, the doctor was killed a week later in a car accident in Damascus. The infection showed no signs of going away. Yima believed that *kirmiz* had special healing properties, so she decided to treat my eyes with it. She put some drops in my eyes and bandaged them to keep the drops in. When she took off the bandages the next day, my eyes had gone white and I was blind.

I was devastated when Mum told me this, but as always, kept my feelings to myself. I could not stop thinking about my eye infection, the American eye doctor, and about Yima and the *kirmiz*. Was this the reason she had always waited on me hand and foot, and hardly let me out of her sight? I could never talk about it with anyone in the family, and they never talked about it with me. I didn't even talk about it with Yola, but sometimes cried about it late at night, when everyone was asleep.

In the meantime, political tensions between Christian and Muslim groups were increasing in Lebanon. By April 1975, there was fighting in the streets between different militias. We often heard gunfire close to our home in central Beirut. Civilians were being captured or killed, and it looked as if a full-scale civil war might break out.

By then, the only ones still living with Mum and Dad in Beirut were Younan, his wife, Olga, their baby boy, and four sisters: Hanne, Margaret, Rima, and me.

Michel and my sisters told us over the phone that Melbourne was a rich and peaceful city with lots of opportunities for work and business. The Australian government, they said, looked after poor people, and even supported old people with a pension when they retired. Surely we would be safe in faraway Australia and never have to flee war or violence again. Mum and Dad decided we should all leave for Melbourne as soon as possible. There was only one problem: they could not get a visa for me because I was blind.

I felt frustrated and guilty that my disability was stopping the family from emigrating to Melbourne. At 23, I too wanted to travel and explore other places, but because I was blind, I could not make my own choices: other people had to decide for me. I craved a life of my own, but had been forced to live in the shade of my parents and siblings. Now my blindness hung like a shadow over all the family, blocking our escape from Lebanon to a life of peace and plenty in Melbourne.

The civil war was becoming more and more violent. There was bombing and gunfire in Haddad in the Maronite part of Beirut, and hundreds of innocent people were being killed in the streets. I would lie in bed shaking with fear as bombs exploded and glass shattered around us. Every night, we had to black out the windows with material so we wouldn't be targeted. One night, we were just about to eat our dinner when there was a loud explosion and the lights went off. The others couldn't eat, but the darkness made no difference to me, so I tucked into my spaghetti while they all went to bed hungry.

By August 1975, full-scale civil war had broken out as the Lebanese national party, backed by Palestinian refugees, tried to take power from the Christian Maronite government. We knew that, as Christians, our lives were in danger.

Then, in the midst of the violence and chaos, something terrible happened. There was a phone call from the Australian embassy asking Dad to go there urgently. They told him that Michel was dead — knocked down by a truck when he was crossing the road in front of the Ford factory.

Dad was in a state of shock but had to think quickly. They needed to leave for Melbourne the next day for the funeral, but Dad knew Mum would collapse when she heard the news, and he feared that she would not be able to get on the plane. He told Mum that it was Yima who had died, not Michel. Dad was crying, and Mum was comforting him, saying that Yima was old, and she'd had a good life, so he shouldn't be too sad now she had passed on. As they left, we were all crying. Rima was howling and holding onto Mum's dress, begging her not to go. I was crying too.

Mum told me I would be responsible for looking after the three younger ones while they were away. Given that I had never been responsible for anything ever before, I was a bit shocked. Now, as the eldest of the four sisters left alone, I was in charge. They took a taxi to the airport, but they almost missed the plane because fighting had broken out around the airport. Dad was anxious about leaving his family in a war zone and told Younan that he should take us back to Syria, where we would be safe.

After they arrived in Melbourne, Dad told Mum the truth — that it was really Michel who had died. She collapsed and screamed at Dad for lying to her. Then she started haemorrhaging from her vagina, and a doctor had to be called.

Back in Beirut, family members were coming to our home, but they were strangely quiet. They had found out from relatives in Melbourne about Michel but had been told not to tell us. Finally, when Antoinette rang to tell us the news, all hell broke loose. Everyone was crying and screaming, friends and family members came running, and for two days the house was filled with people sobbing and wailing. We couldn't believe that Michel, our loved eldest brother, was gone — just like that.

Sherine was most affected, because she was closest to him. Even now, 50 years later, she is still broken-hearted about his death. Whenever she goes to church and hears the priest chanting, she thinks of Michel and can't stop herself from crying.

A week after he died, we received another big shock: Mum and Dad decided to stay in Melbourne and not come back to Beirut at all. They were going to leave us four sisters on our own in Beirut. However, they had a very good reason. Mr Whitlam, the then Prime Minister of Australia, had announced an amnesty: anyone who arrived before or during 1975 on visitors' visas could apply for permanent residency. If my parents didn't stay, they would probably not be allowed to return later. It was the only chance for us all to get to Australia eventually. Dad applied again for visas for the rest of the family, but I was again rejected.

They had only taken a few clothes with them, but for some reason Mum had packed her favourite possession: a brass samovar that stands about 30 centimetres tall. You put hot coals in a tray on the bottom to heat water, which you then poured from a long, curved spout. Instead of a lid there was a small teapot on the top, so tea could be kept warm. I was with her when she saw it in a shop window in Beirut and fell in love with it. She handed it to me so I could feel it, then she bought it for 25 lira. Perhaps she took the samovar with her to Melbourne to give to Michel, or because she knew they might stay there and may not ever return home. Today, the samovar has pride of place in the lounge room, and it is the only memento we have of our life in the Middle East.

Dad sent Younan money and detailed instructions on how to get us out of Beirut, so we packed a few clothes and left all the family's belongings at the church to be given to poor people. It was a sad, confusing time. So much had happened in just one month. Michel was dead, and I did not know when I would see Mum, Dad, or Yima again, or whether I would ever come back to Beirut once we had left. I was stranded with my three younger sisters, without our parents or older sisters to look after us, and we had to escape from a horrible civil war. Maybe I could go to America and be with Nimo in Chicago if Australia didn't want me. That was my dream. America seemed like a more glamorous place to live in than Australia.

We said goodbye to our home in Haddad and set off for Syria in September 1975, two weeks after Michel had died. There was just one positive thing: we were going to live with Mum's younger sister, Yonia, and her husband, Samuel, in Ras al Ain, a town in the north east, not far from Hasakah and Tel Wardiyat. I knew Yonia and Samuel were easy-going and laughed a lot, so I had a good feeling about going to stay with them.

5
Ras al Ain:
The Healing Spring

I felt a wave of relief as the taxi crossed the border from war-torn Lebanon into peaceful Syria. At Damascus, we took a bus for the overnight trip back north through Aleppo and Homs to Hasakah, then another bus to our old village, just half an hour further on.

It was nine years since we had left there, and everyone came out to welcome us. We stayed in our house with Mum's cousin Ushana and his family, who had taken it over when we went to Beirut. The house was the same as I remembered it. Without sewerage, running water, or electricity, it seemed primitive in comparison with our apartment in Beirut. We had emotional reunions with friends and family members. People sat with us to cry for Michel, and everyone invited us for lunches and dinners.

After a week, we caught the bus to our final destination
— the town of Ras al Ain, right on the border with
Turkey. Hanne, Margaret, Rima, and I were to stay with
Aunt Yonia and Uncle Samuel, while Younan and his wife
and baby stayed with relatives in Hasakah.

Ras al Ain means 'Head of the Spring'. It's the name
of a famous hot mineral spring that flows into the Khabur
River before it joins the Euphrates. The spring smells like
rotten eggs, but people come from far and wide to bathe
in it because of its special healing powers. One day, they
took me there, but I stayed as far away as I could from the
awful smell. I knew it was an historic, even supernatural
place, but I never wanted to go back.

Yonia and Samuel welcomed us into their home as
if we were long-lost daughters. They had a single-storey
house with a big kitchen, bathroom, indoor toilet, and
three large bedrooms: one for the boys, one for the girls,
and one for them. Another room had been converted into
a small clinic where Samuel, a general practitioner, could
see his patients.

Samuel worked long hours attending his patients, who
were mainly Muslim. Nearly every day he would be off on
home visits, woken up at all hours of the night by husbands
who would take him home to deliver babies when their
wives were in labour. He was over 70, but was still working

because he loved it, and often treated sick people for free. He didn't have a car and had to be driven whenever he went on a home visit. Of course, he treated us as well, and gave us medicines whenever we needed them.

Yonia was his second wife. His first wife had died, leaving him with a small daughter. After he and Yonia married, they had seven children, who were then aged from three to 16 years of age. Nevertheless, they could not do enough for us. Now their family had grown to 11, four boys and seven girls, but this time I was the eldest.

On the day we arrived, they had beds ready for us in the girls' bedroom. As in every family home, the mattresses were stacked against the walls during the day and put on the floor at night, so we just joined in with our cousins. It was like suddenly getting three new sisters, and the seven of us would talk and giggle every night before we went to sleep.

Every second day, Yonia kneaded dough, left it to rise, then baked delicious, yeasty-smelling loaves of bread. At mealtimes she would make two big casseroles, one with rice or pasta and one with meat, lentils, or chickpeas, and different vegetables. Everything was served with salads and her home-made yoghurt.

There was a lively atmosphere in the family. Yonia and Samuel talked about life and politics more than Mum and Dad, so I learned a lot just by listening. Living with them, I felt more relaxed than I did at home. No-one was watching me, protecting me, or telling me what to do, and they treated me not as a blind person but as an equal. We didn't go out much, as there was nowhere to go, but I didn't mind.

One major anxiety was weighing me down, though — my responsibility for the welfare and good behaviour of my three younger sisters. I felt completely unprepared to be the one in charge. I laid down the law and made them stay home all day with me, anxious about what might happen if they went out. As Assyrians, we didn't cover our heads like Muslim girls did, so we felt vulnerable, especially as we were in a predominantly Muslim area.

I worried constantly that they would not behave themselves. How could I know what they were up to when I couldn't see them? If we were sitting together in a room, I always made them tell me where they were, so I could be sure they were actually there. Sometimes our cousins teased me, telling me my sisters had disappeared and nobody knew where they were. I didn't get upset about the teasing, though, because I knew it was all in fun.

The way I coped was to be strict and controlling, just like Yima had been. Because of all the stories I had heard about Muslim men looking out for non-Muslim girls,

I forbade them to go down the street to the local shop. Instead, I made them write down anything they wanted on a piece of paper and give it to one of the boys to buy. Sometimes they rebelled against me. Rima was the most rebellious, and kept on pestering me to let her go out. One day, when she would not take no for an answer, I grabbed her, whacked her on the bum, and that was that. We still laugh about it.

I came to love Yonia and Samuel not just as aunt and uncle but as real friends. They never complained about having four extra mouths to feed and made us feel like special guests. Samuel would call me to get up early every morning to have coffee with him, and we would sit down and talk about anything and everything. We had a special connection. He would ask me about my blindness, and say what a tragedy it was that I had been blinded by *kirmiz*.

Yonia was always laughing and joking, and sometimes played tricks on us. One day, when Hanne and Yonia were doing the washing together, Yonia said, 'Go and tell Marie that I don't want you to stay here anymore. Tell her I said you all have to go because it's too much for me … just tell her that and see what she says.'

Hanne came up to me, all distressed, and told me what Yonia had said. I thought, *Oh, my God, now what are we going to do?*

I said to Hanne, 'Don't say anything, and we'll get a taxi tomorrow back to Tel Wardiyat. We can stay with our cousins there.' Hanne said, 'No, we have to go back to Lebanon! I'm going to kill myself!' I started crying, then Yonia came rushing up and put her arms around me: 'I'm so sorry, it's OK, I was only joking, I was just trying you out. Of course I want you all to stay here! I love you all!'

Perhaps she wanted to clear the air in case we were worried that we were not wanted? It was a strange trick to play on us, but soon everything was back to normal, and I never doubted that we were loved and welcome.

One day, in August the following year, Rima looked out of the window and called out, 'Look, there's a lady wearing black coming along the street ... it's my sister Sherine, I can see her!' It was true; suddenly, Sherine walked into the house. The others started jumping on her, hugging her and crying. Rima said, 'Why did you come here? Are you going to take us back?' 'Yes', said Sherine. 'I've come to take you back to Athens, and after that we'll all go to Australia.' Rima was beside herself with joy and would not let go of Sherine, who was wearing black because we were still in mourning for Michel. We all wore black, except for Rima, who was too young.

Unknown to us, Dad had asked Sherine to come over from Greece and take us to live with her in Athens, while we waited for our Australian visas to come through. She had flown from Athens to Damascus, and then come by bus to Ras al Ain to collect us.

In a few days, we were packed and ready to go. Everyone was crying. Samuel was sobbing like a little kid. 'Thank you for the wonderful time we had together,' he said. 'I know I'll never see you again.' We never did see him again, as he died about two years later.

I'll always be grateful for my year with Yonia, Samuel, and their family. With them, I hadn't been the quiet blind girl who did what she was told and had nothing much to say. Instead, I had been with people who accepted me as an adult and made me feel special, so I came alive in their presence. My responsibility for my sisters had made me feel mature and respected.

To this day, my aunt and cousins from Ras al Ain are my closest friends within our extended family. Some are living in Melbourne, and they often say that it is thanks to me that they made the happy choice to come and live here. Yonia, now in her late 70s, lives with three of her sons and two daughters in Germany. I often chat with her on the phone, and we still laugh a lot.

I never bathed in the mineral waters of Ras al Ain, but all the same, a kind of healing had taken place inside of me. My Ras al Ain family had given me a year of friendship and laughter, bringing me confidence and hope for the future.

Sherine, Hanne, Margaret, Rima, and I once again took the gruelling ten-hour bus trip to Damascus. Sherine looked for a taxi driver who would take us across the border to Jounieh, just north of Beirut, where we would catch a boat to Cyprus. She was looking for a driver without a beard, because a man with a beard might be a Muslim extremist, one of the bad ones.

We found a friendly, clean-shaven driver who was happy to take the five of us into Lebanon. He said, however, that it would be too dangerous for him to drive to Beirut because of the fighting. Instead, we would take a detour, and go directly to Jounieh. Sherine sat in the front with the driver, with a basket of sandwiches, fruit, and water for the two-hour trip, while the four younger sisters were crammed in the back.

When they told me that we had crossed the border into Lebanon, I started to feel scared. After a short while, the car stopped. A soldier standing on the side of the road had flagged us down. He said he wanted us to take him to another army camp further along the road. The driver refused. Then the man stood in front of the taxi, opened a bag, and pulled out a hand grenade. I couldn't see what was happening, of course, but the others whispered everything to me.

'Let me get in the car or I'll blow it up right now,' he said. We went very quiet, thinking we might die any second. The driver said, 'Please, they are girls — you can't just blow us up!' The man said, 'OK, I'll let you go, but when you come back, I'll be waiting for you and I'll fix you up then.'

Sherine opened the window and said to the soldier, 'It's not his fault — he's just a driver. We are sisters, and we have to get to Jounieh. What do you want?' He said, 'I haven't eaten for three days, I'm thirsty, and I haven't slept. I just need to get from here to the next army base so I can eat and get some rest.'

She said, 'OK, we'll take you. I'll sit in the back and you can sit in the front.' So Sherine squashed into the back seat with us, while he got in the front and wolfed down the sandwiches, fruit, and water that she gave him. When he got out half an hour later, he apologised, thanked us, and said how desperate he had been.

At last we arrived at the house Sherine had rented for us in Jounieh. It took ten days for Sherine to organise visas for us to go to Greece. Finally, on Tuesday 15 August 1976, we set sail for Athens.

6
Athens: Learning Greek with Heraklea

The overnight voyage in a small ferry from Lebanon to Cyprus was my first time at sea. We took our places on wooden seats in the open air. I felt the ocean rolling beneath me, smelled salty sea air, and heard seabirds crying.

But the waves got bigger and bigger, and a fierce storm blew up. The voyage turned into a nightmare. We huddled together, vomiting and drenched with sea spray. I could hear plastic flapping in the wind and men shouting to each other as the crew tried to put up tarpaulins to protect the passengers. But they gave up because the wind was too strong. For hours we clung to each other in the dark, terrified, wet, and sick. At about 4am, the waves began to die down. The captain announced that the boat had become lost in the storm, but now they had found their bearings and we would be in Larnaca in a few hours.

At Larnaca they lowered a gangplank onto the wharf, but it was swaying from side to side, and there were no handrails for me to hold onto. The others walked down onto the wharf, but I refused to budge, certain I would lose my balance and fall into the water. Then a kind man came to my rescue. He told me to stand behind him, hold onto his waist, push my toes against the back of his shoes and slide my feet forward when he took each step. We must have looked funny shuffling down the gangplank together with our shoes touching, but I didn't care. I was safe. On dry land at last, I clung to my sisters as the ground rocked up and down for a minute or two, just like the sea.

Then we had another shock. When Sherine showed our visas to the Greek immigration officers, they said she was the only one who would be allowed into the country. The rest of us would have to go back to Lebanon because she was not our legal guardian. Sherine begged and pleaded, saying that our parents were in Australia, and she couldn't take us back to Syria because she had her own young family to look after in Athens, and that we had nowhere to go in Lebanon. Eventually, they gave us visas and let us into Larnaca, where we got on another ferry for the three-day voyage to Athens.

This ferry was huge, like a four-storey building with comfortable seats. I stood on the deck, holding onto the rail, and looked out at the sea. I could just make out the dark green of the waves and clumps of white foam. Hanne told me there were dolphins swimming alongside the boat and described them to me. I tried to imagine them and thought they must be half fish, half human, like mermaids. Little Rima, desperately missing Mum, said she wished she could be like Jonah and jump into the mouth of a whale, so it could take her straight to Melbourne and cough her up onto the beach there.

On the last night a wind blew up, the sea heaved, and I was seasick again. The boat docked at the island of Rhodes for a few hours, and I heard trucks being driven on and off before we sailed out to sea again. Then, in the middle of the night, the ship's engines suddenly went silent, and there was a screaming noise as anchors were dropped into the ocean. Everything stayed quiet for several hours — we had no idea why — then the engines throbbed back to life, the anchors came up, and we continued on our way. At last, Hanne and Margaret told me they could see the lights of Athens on the horizon.

It was still dark when a taxi took us to the small house where Sherine's husband, Saleba, and their four children were waiting. With the addition of us four girls, their family had suddenly grown to ten. We all slept in the one bedroom, the children two or three to a bed, and we were happy. With Sherine now in charge, I no longer had to be responsible for my three younger sisters. Sherine and Saleba were lovely, and they took me with them whenever they went out. We all looked forward to being reunited with Mum, Dad, and Yima in Melbourne, and spoke about little else.

Once again, we were in a close-knit Assyrian community within a mainstream community that spoke a different language. Quite a few friends and relatives who had fled from Iraq in the 1930s or from the civil war in Lebanon were there, so we felt at home. Grandmother Sarah, her two sons, her daughter-in-law and grandchildren lived nearby, and there were several cousins who had been born there and spoke perfect Greek. Every Sunday, we got together at a little church that had been set up by an Assyrian priest in a rented room. The candlelight, prayers, chanting, and incense brought the Holy Spirit into that small room. Church took us away from our everyday problems and brought us close to God and the mystery of creation.

Dad sent money from Australia to help support us. Every time our cousins came to visit, they would bring bags of groceries — tins of chickpeas, tuna, tomato paste, cheese, and butter. My cousin Lazarus, who was born in Greece, came once a month. Each time he did, he would secretly put folded notes of money into my hand. When I protested, he would say, 'No, you are here in place of your mother, so it's really for her.'

I got over my fear of being in a new country with a new language and fell a little bit in love with Greece. The summer sky seemed bluer and the air had a cleaner smell than in Syria, perhaps because of the sea. The fruit-and-vegetable market had sounds and smells that were new to me, and there was a delicious aroma of Greek food and home-baked bread wafting from neighbours' kitchens. On hot summer days we stayed inside, not doing much, then in the cool of the evening went out to walk, joining other families who came out for their nightly stroll. Greek people were kind and good-natured, especially when we struggled to communicate in shops. Greek neighbours gave us furniture, including four beds and an icebox. Every two days someone had to go out and buy a big block of ice to keep our food fresh.

Boredom was still my worst enemy. There was nothing for me to do during the day except go downstairs, pack and unpack, pack and unpack my small suitcase of belongings. I spent most days sitting in my corner listening to whatever was going on around me, as I had always done. The days drifted by, and I had no idea if I would ever get to Australia or where I would end up.

After three months, visas arrived for Hanne, Margaret, and Rima. I was overjoyed when they flew off to Melbourne, because I knew how much they needed Mum and Dad. Again, I had been knocked back for a visa, but I took it philosophically. I missed my three younger sisters, but they would be happy, and that was what mattered the most. I would survive whatever happened and might even finish up living my secret dream in America.

Every day, before we went out, Sherine and Saleba would inspect me to make sure I looked smart and tidy. My dress, shoes, and hair had to be perfect. They were proud of me and taught me to take pride in my appearance. One day, Saleba came home with a beautiful summer dress for me, brown with white lace around the neckline. I felt elegant in it and started taking an interest in clothes and fashion. Knowing I was well-groomed gave me confidence — I felt good about myself if I knew I looked good, even if I couldn't see myself.

I loved their children, especially the twins, Peter and Paul, and my darling niece Sonia. Eleven-year-old Sonia took me walking, my arm through hers, when we went out in the evenings. She was like a small, chatty friend at my side, always describing where we were and pointing out steps, branches, or obstacles I might bump into.

After a year, Sherine and Saleba got visas and were preparing to go to Australia. My brother Younan would be the last of the Younan family, apart from me, who had not gone to Australia or America, so it was his job to stay with me in Athens until my visa came. We moved into a new house and his wife, Olga, became my friend. We would get up at eight every morning while Younan was still asleep, sit together in the freezing cold kitchen, chat and drink coffee. Younan was ten years older than me and took on a parental role, watching over me the way Yima used to do. Sometimes I got fed up with his advice and warnings, but I knew it was because he felt responsible for me and was doing his best.

Heraklea, our lovely landlady, lived next door. Every day, she would call me to her home for a sandwich and coffee, and give me Nutella rolls to take home for my little nephew.

With Heraklea as my friend, life took on new meaning. She took it on herself to teach me Greek by putting food and other objects into my hands, naming them, and acting out simple phrases. I quickly picked up the meanings, repeating the words and phrases and asking Lazarus, my Greek-speaking cousin, to explain those I didn't understand. Soon he was teaching me as well, and in a few months, I could buy things in the shops and speak a little bit of Greek as my third language. My Greek lessons were always accompanied by food. Every Wednesday and Friday, Heraklea cooked fish and invited me to eat it with her. When the mouth-watering smell of frying fish came floating from her kitchen window, I knew it was time to go there.

Heraklea was deeply religious. She went to the Greek Orthodox church on Sundays and three times a day on weekdays, at 6am, midday, and 6pm, when she would light incense and pray. She would ask God to bless all people, not just her own family. She cared about people in every country in the world. She was the one person I could talk to about how I felt, deep down, about being locked out of Australia and away from my parents because of being blind. I cried when I told her about my fear that Younan and Olga would go to Australia and leave me on my own in Athens. I was much too proud to share those feelings with anyone in the family. Heraklea would say, 'Don't worry, you'll go to Australia sometime soon.' She asked me to call her 'Mum' and told me that if I couldn't go to Australia, I could live with her. She would send me to a hostel for the blind, bring me home to stay with her every weekend, and look after me like a daughter. But I never gave up hope, and every week or so I would use her phone to call the Australian embassy to see if my visa had come through.

One night in November, a fierce electrical storm exploded over Athens. Rain poured down for hours, the electricity went off, and water began flowing down our street. Younan was away, and Olga and I were terrified. Olga wanted to run to Sherine's house, but I said, 'No, it's too dangerous, we might drown!' It's lucky we didn't, as many people did drown that night, trying to escape the floodwaters that washed through Athens. Eventually, Heraklea called us to go upstairs at her house until the water went down. At Sherine's house it was worse: she found everything was ruined when she went downstairs and water came to her waist. Olga still reminds me that I saved her life and mine by refusing to go out on the night of the flood.

A few weeks after the flood, Sherine and her family left for Melbourne, while Younan, Olga, and I continued our quiet life in Athens. Every day, I went to Heraklea's house to talk, eat snacks, and learn more Greek. Sometimes she gave me hot spinach water to drink, saying it was good for me. The spinach water had the taste of good health and Heraklea's loving soul.

After waiting for more than a year, I began to feel depressed. Every time a plane flew over, I would say, 'I don't care where that plane is going, I just want to be on it!' Then one day, in January 1978, I rang the embassy and there *was* news … My brother-in-law Peter had sponsored me, and my visa was waiting to be picked up! I hung up the phone with a big grin on my face. Heraklea started crying, and said, 'Oh darling, I love you. I'm glad to see you go, but I know I'll never see you again!'

She insisted on cooking a special dinner the day before I left, and asked me what my favourite Greek dish was. I said her moussaka, as it was the most delicious thing I had ever tasted. She invited Younan and Olga to my farewell dinner, but they thought it would be better for Heraklea and me to be alone so we could speak Greek at our last meal together. I said sad farewells to Heraklea, Olga, and Younan and prepared myself for the flight to Australia and reunion at last with the rest of my family.

On a cold day at the end of February 1978, I was packed and ready to go. Sarah, now in her 80s, was to accompany me on the flight to Melbourne to see her two daughters,

Mum and my aunt Susan. Sarah's son, my uncle Andreas, took us to the airport with a Greek-speaking cousin to help. When he went to check us in, Sarah kept going off on her own, so I used my special foot-sliding way of walking around the airport to try to find her. Later, a man came up and said to my cousin in Greek, 'Who is this girl? I'd like to take care of her on the flight.' He said to me, 'My name is Thanassi, and I'm on your plane. From this minute, I'm going to be your brother and you're going to be my sister. I'll look after you. Don't worry about a thing.'

Sarah and I were nervous, never having been on a plane before. When Thanassi led me inside the plane and found us our seats, it was like walking into a big house with hundreds of people packed into it. Sarah was too scared to sit near a window, so Thanassi took the window seat while I was in the middle, with Sarah on my other side. As the plane took off, he told me what he could see out the window — houses, hills, sea, islands, clouds, and then just the dark night. I tried to interpret for Sarah, but she said she didn't want to know about it.

Thanassi was good fun and treated me like his best friend. I couldn't understand everything he said in Greek and often had to ask him to repeat himself, but we got by. When meals came, he told me what was on the menu, and cut up my food so I could eat it with a fork and spoon. He filled in my forms and even took me to the toilet. An air hostess came too, but he waited outside and clasped his hands behind his back to lead me back to my seat. Sarah slept most of the time and hardly said anything all the way. Thanks to Thanassi, the flight was easy, but I couldn't sleep with the exciting prospect of meeting all my family in just a few hours.

We arrived in Melbourne at about 3am. Thanassi came with us for a short while before continuing on to Sydney. He found our cases, put them on a trolley, found a Greek-speaking attendant to look after us, and said goodbye. I hardly knew what to say to him, my friend of less than 24 hours. When I thanked him, he said, 'My Dad is very sick, so I have to do something good for him and for God.'

He gave me his business card, and we promised to keep in touch.

The attendant took our passports and led me through immigration while Sarah followed behind with the trolley. We walked for several minutes then I heard a door opening ... suddenly Antoinette was there, hugging me and sobbing. Mum threw her arms around me, and Dad and Peter hugged me. I was speechless, as if in a strange dream. Was this Australia at last?

I walked into a wave of warm air, a pleasant surprise after Athens' chilly winter. That was when I found out that the seasons in Australia are opposite to the seasons in the northern hemisphere. Nobody had told me about the seasons, and that the earth was round and went around the sun. When we got into Peter's car, everyone suddenly went quiet. I felt like a zombie, choked with feelings that were too strong to be let out.

Yima and my sisters were still in bed when we got to our family home in Reservoir. Rosa, Michel's widow, came out to greet us and said, 'This is my daughter, Elizabeth.' When I touched my four-year-old niece for the first time, my tears flowed: tears of relief and joy at being reunited with my family; tears of sorrow for Michel who was no longer with us; and tears of love for this little girl who had no father. Then Dad started crying and everyone else joined in. It was the most beautiful moment of my life.

Later that afternoon, I found my way into the backyard and stood for a while in the hot sun. What would my new country be like? How would I learn the language? How would I be?

7
Melbourne:
The Promised Land

I was blown away by Mum and Dad's house.

Number 2 Leech Street Reservoir was a large brick home, with a rose garden in front and a vegetable garden at the back. It was like a palace compared to the houses I knew in Syria and Greece, with a modern kitchen, tiled bathroom, and a big, comfortable lounge room. For once, I could walk around without having to squeeze my way past people and furniture all the time.

Thirteen of us fitted in quite comfortably. Mum, Dad, and Sarah slept in one room, Rosa and her three daughters in another, while Hanne, Margaret, Rima, and I were in the third bedroom, and Yima shared a small room with Evette.

Yima was 100 now, and was like a tiny, frail skeleton.

She rarely spoke but she knew what was going on around her. The doctor said she was in perfect health, just fading away with old age. She was pleased to see me, but she said very little, as if she was only half there.

Mum proudly showed me around the house. She led me down four steps into the backyard so I could touch everything and get my bearings. I could see the bright-green lawn and smell its fresh, grassy smell. A cement path led to the clothesline, which was made of iron and went around in a circle. Mum showed me how to swing it around and wind it up and down with a handle. The rubbish bins were amazing. Back home, rubbish bins stank because they were small and over-flowing but here, they were big plastic bins with hinged lids, and wheels for moving them on to the street on collection days.

I knelt down and felt the vegies in Dad's vegie garden: tomatoes, cucumber, eggplant, peppers, parsley, mint, and coriander. Growing vegetables and fruit trees in our own backyard was another luxury. In Tel Wardiyat, our vegetable garden was a 15-minute walk away, and I had only been there once or twice. I loved being able to go outside and smell the herbs and tomatoes, and touch the plants to see how fast they were growing.

Everything in the house and garden was safe, clean, and orderly. I woke every morning to bird song and the quiet hum of cars driving up and down the street — not like the noisy backstreets I was used to. A sense of relief and well-being flowed through me: *thank God I'm here at last in my new country with all my family around me!*

When they arrived in 1975, Dad was 65 and Mum was 51. Neither of them learned English or had any contact with English-speaking Australians. But they loved Australia. Dad liked telling people that even though he had worked all his life in Syria and Lebanon, the Australian government paid his pension. That made him proud to be here. But he never worked again or drove a car. His work now was to tend his vegetables and roses and do the household shopping. He wrote his weekly shopping list with careful attention to detail, asking everyone what they needed or wanted him to buy, and once a week Rosa or Janet drove him to Victoria Market. Every day, he would work away in his garden with the same care: weeds were never allowed to show their heads, and everyone commented on how glorious the roses were — bright red, deep burgundy, yellow, orange, pink, and white. The rose perfume would fill the front garden and waft down the street. I put rose petals in a bowl and ran my hands through them to feel their soft texture and release their fragrance. Mum made me a small cloth bag, which I filled with the dried petals and kept in my clothes drawer.

We had flywire screens to keep insects out, but my moth phobia was as bad as ever. If a moth flew into the house, I had to go straight to bed and put my head under the blankets. Sometimes I dreamed about moths and woke up screaming.

Mum and Dad were happy together and talked about everything between themselves. After 40 years of marriage, Dad would say how much he loved Mum and what a wonderful woman she was. Every year, he would buy her an expensive bunch of long-stemmed red roses for Mothers' Day. She always complained that they cost too much, but they made her happy all the same.

Five of their ten daughters were still living at home: Hanne, Margaret, Evette, Rima, and me. Michel's widow, our sister-in-law Rosa, was also living with us, along with her three daughters.

My older sisters Nimo and Mona were settled with their families in Chicago and often talked on the phone with us. Antoinette, Peter, and their children were living in a flat above their fish-and-chip shop in bayside Mornington. Sherine and Janet lived nearby in Reservoir and called in nearly every day. My sisters had found good jobs. Sherine, Evette, and Janet worked at the Visyboard cardboard factory in Reservoir, and Hanne and Margaret worked at the Nestlé chocolate factory in Campbellfield.

Rima was still at high school. Our brother Younan was still in Greece with his family, planning to join us in Melbourne as soon as he could.

Rosa never worked and never remarried. Her daughters and the other grandchildren did well at the local school. They were the ones who brought English language and Aussie culture into the family.

A few weeks after I arrived, they told me what I already knew: that Yima was weak with old age and would not live for much longer. I often thought about what a wonderful woman she had been, despite so much tragedy and hardship in her early life. I still agonised about the guilt she must have been living with because of making me go blind. One day, I went into her room and said, 'Yima, they gave me an operation, and I can see now.' She said, 'I don't believe you. You're only saying that to make me happy because I'm dying. I know you will never be able to see!'

Shortly after I arrived in Melbourne, Antoinette and Peter asked if I could live with them in Mornington, as they wanted me to be part of their family. I gladly moved into their flat above the shop. They had five girls and a boy, their oldest girl having already married and left home. I shared a room with two of their girls, Helen and Maria, two lovely nieces whom I had never met before. We ate lots of fish and chips, and I was on top of the world.

When we received word that Yima had passed away, we drove straight to Melbourne. The whole family was weeping. Yima had been the centre and strength of the family for so many years, and had taught us how to care for each other and other people.

Back at Mornington, my nieces were always asking me what I wanted, or what they could do for me. One day, they took me for my first ever walk along a beach. I could just see the blue of the sea and light-brown sand. I heard the gentle splashing of the waves and felt the sand squishing between my toes. I dipped my hands into the sea to feel the water washing to and fro. It was a moment of joyfulness in my new country.

But I still had nothing to do, and the boredom was killing me. Sometimes I thought I would die from having nothing to do and very little to think about.

Then one day, Antoinette met a customer, a blind man called Ivan Molloy, whose job it was to meet and support other blind people. He told us he had lost his sight at the age of 11 when a boy threw a stone into his eye.

Ivan told us about a Day Care Centre for blind people called the 'George Vowell Centre', not far away in Mt Eliza, and arranged for me to go there. Antoinette took me, and they invited me to learn basket-weaving for two days a week. Soon I was weaving baskets and getting to know some of the other people at the centre. But I found it hard because I didn't know enough English to communicate. Being blind *and* not speaking the language was like having a double obstacle that prevented me from making friends. I had picked up Greek quickly with Heraklea as my personal language teacher and friend, but here I couldn't learn English in the same way.

One day, Ivan gave me a braille watch and told me I could tell the time with it. This was an exciting prospect — it was the first time I heard about braille, and I had never thought that I'd be able to tell the time on my own. It took me a few weeks to learn how to use the watch. When you opened it, you could feel the position of the hands and the 12 raised points around the outside that represented the numbers. My nieces Helen and Maria and nephew George were my teachers. George got an apple and cut it into four pieces, to help explain that an hour was divided into four 15-minute pieces, which were the quarter hours. Then he got me to feel the four quarters on the watch and each of the numbers that made up 12 hours. Every day, the three of them sat down with me and gave me a lesson. Then I had to remember that there were four lots of three hours every 12 hours, and two lots of

12 hours every 24 hours. Soon I could tell the time and went around asking people, 'Can I tell you the time?' I remembered that my grandmothers could only tell the time by looking at the sun, and I was grateful.

Antoinette also introduced me to a Greek man, Kyriakos, who delivered seafood to their shop. Kyriakos spoke with me in Greek and insisted that I go to stay with him and his wife in Altona. I refused at first, as I hardly knew them and was terrified. But Antoinette made me go, and I have never regretted it. Kyriakos and his wife, Connie, are lovely people, and were my first real friends in Australia. Every time I went there, they would sit around the table and talk. Sometimes they would sing, clap their hands, and do Greek dancing in the kitchen.

Connie would take me shopping and sometimes bought me clothes. We used to go to the hairdressers together to have our hair done. One day, we came back with our hair set in smart hairstyles. I said I didn't want to go to bed that night in case I ruined my new hairdo. Kyriakos said, 'Why don't you just take your head off and leave it on the bedside table overnight?' That night I arranged three pillows so I could sleep on my stomach, with my head poking down into the hole between the pillows. The next morning, when they told me that my hair looked perfect, I told them I had taken my head off to sleep, and put it back on again when I got up.

Ivan Molloy often called in to see how I was going and ask what other support I needed. One day, he told me something amazing — that it might be possible for me to have an operation to get my sight back.

In July 1978, Ivan and Antoinette took me to a doctor who referred me to an eye specialist at the Eye and Ear Hospital. The specialist said that my corneas were damaged and that I had glaucoma. That was the first time I heard the word 'glaucoma'. He said that a corneal transplant might restore my sight, and a date was set for 10 September. I could hardly believe it. I lived every day in hope, while trying not to get too excited in case the operation failed.

Before the operation, Antoinette's children taught me some English words I would need while I was in hospital. They taught me 'I want to go to the toilet', 'I'm in pain', 'I'm scared', 'I'm worried', and some names of foods. Connie and Kyriakos took me to Southlands and bought me a lovely burgundy dressing gown and new nighties to wear in hospital. Everyone was thrilled with the possibility that I might soon be able to see. I moved back to be with Mum and Dad in Reservoir before I had the operation.

The tenth of September came around at last. Before I went into the operating theatre, I asked them, with Antoinette interpreting, who had donated their corneas after they had died. They told me it was a 16-year-old boy who had died in a car accident. I felt sad for him and his family, and deeply grateful for his gift to me.

I woke up with pads on my eyes and could not resist lifting one of them and having a little peek, but the nurse caught me and said I would have to wait. After three days they took off the bandages. I could see a few dim shapes. I saw a cup, but I found it hard to relate what I saw to the idea of a cup that I had in my head from feeling it. I could see a black square that I knew was my transistor radio on my bed, and could also see curtains on the window. I said to myself, 'Bit by bit, I will be able to see.'

When the nurse came in with a meal, she said, 'Here's your lunch: meat is at 12 o'clock, potato at two o'clock, and vegetables at nine o'clock.' I couldn't work out what on earth was going on. Did Australians have to eat the different foods at different times? Terrified of doing the wrong thing, I only ate my meat, and thought I had to wait until the proper times to eat the potatoes and vegetables. When the nurse came back and I told her why I hadn't finished my lunch, she explained that she had meant the position of the foods on the plate, and we both had a good laugh.

Every day, the doctor came around and asked me if I had a headache. When I said 'No,' he would say, 'That's good news.' For four days all went well, then, on the fifth day, I suddenly had a bad headache, and had to take some tablets. The doctor said, 'Oh no, that's terrible, that's really bad luck.' I knew from the tone of his voice that it was all over. The headache was caused by my eyeballs swelling, and that meant that the corneas were being rejected.

In 1980, they tried for a second time to give me a corneal transplant, but that too failed. A few years later, they tried for a third and final time. With each operation I went through the same cycle of hope and disappointment. By then, my retinas were so badly damaged by the pressure from my eyeballs that over the next few years I lost the ability to see even the tiny bits of colour that I could see before.

Also in 1980, Janet got engaged to an Assyrian man called Sam, and a small wedding was planned. I was invited, but the mark in my heart was still there, telling me that I shouldn't go because I was blind. Weddings were supposed to be happy occasions, I said to myself, and I didn't want people to feel sad because they saw me there or feel as if they had to look after me.

Five years later, Hanne got married to an Assyrian man who was also called Sam. Again, I decided not to go to the wedding. This time my sister Evette, four years younger than me, stayed home to keep me company. Evette was very independent and never wanted to get married, having turned down several offers from eligible Assyrian men. Evette and I were on the same wavelength and talked about anything and everything.

Around 1983, Mum flew to Chicago to visit Mona, Nimo, and their families, taking 19-year-old Rima with her. While they were there, Rima fell in love with an Assyrian man called Jack, and they became engaged almost immediately. The next year, Mum and Rima flew over for the wedding. Rima and Jack settled in Phoenix, Arizona, where they set up a travel agency and had three children.

Of the ten Younan sisters, three had settled in the USA and seven of us were in Melbourne: Antoinette, Sherine Janet, Hanne, Evette, Margaret, and me, along with our sister-in-law Rosa, who was really another sister.

After I moved back to Reservoir with Mum and Dad, Ivan organised for me to go to the Coburg Day Centre for blind people, so I could meet other blind people and do handicrafts. For three years, from 1982 to 1985, I went one day a week. Again, I struggled to make friends with native-born Australians because my English was not up to it, and I felt like an outsider. I made just one lovely friend, an Albanian woman called Millie, who was losing her sight because of diabetes. She spoke very basic English, like I did, so we could communicate on the same level. Millie and I always sat together, and we became inseparable. Whenever we went on excursions in the bus, the staff would joke that we were really two halves of one person.

Our days were spent weaving baskets and making pots or small figures out of clay, and sometimes they took us on excursions in the minibus. The zoo was my favourite place to visit. The staff would describe the various animals while we stood outside the cages and took in their sounds and smells. I was thrilled by the roar of lions and the deep growling of tigers.

One day, they took us into the butterfly house. I would never have gone in had I known the meaning of the word 'butterfly', which in Assyrian is the same word as 'moth'. As soon as I felt that dreaded soft fluttering around my hair I realised where I was. I freaked out completely and said, 'Get me out of here!' When I got back home, I felt like throwing myself in the washing machine. Everyone laughed when I told them I had been inside a moth house by mistake.

Staff members at the Day Centre would take me into the kitchen and teach me the names of things such as 'fridge', 'teapot' and 'milk'. Bit by bit, I began to grasp the meanings of common English words. I also enjoyed crafts, and found I was good at them. In 1982, I even won first prize at a local show for a lampshade base I had modelled out of clay.

Meantime, my friend Millie became seriously ill with diabetes, and her blood sugar levels were out of control. She was weaving a basket as a gift for her granddaughter when she said to me, 'If I die, will you finish this for me?' I said, 'Don't talk like that; you're not going to die!' Soon after, she went to Albania to visit her family, and she had a stroke at the airport on the way back. She was rushed to hospital and died the next day. So I did finish the basket for her granddaughter, and Mum put in a doll dressed with clothes she had crocheted. Millie's son shed tears when we gave it to them.

Mum and Dad were contented, but their contentment was tinged with sadness. It was hard for Dad to be without work and to no longer have the companionship and respect of workmates. They were isolated from the Australian community, and their lives were narrowly contained. Mum never got over losing Michel. She never let us have a Christmas tree on Christmas day as a symbol that, having lost him, our happiness would never be complete. Even though they still had each other, 11 children, their partners, and dozens of grandchildren, they held onto their grief and remained loyal to his memory. Perhaps the loss of Michel came to symbolise all the loved ones they had lost over the years when they were refugees travelling from country to country, and for that reason he could never be forgotten.

I too had a layer of sadness despite being with my family in this rich, peaceful country. I began to think that, like Mum and Dad, I would never really feel at home in Australia. Why should I struggle to learn such a difficult language as English when I had nobody to speak it to? Even though I loved my family, I was dependent on them for everything, while hungering for other relationships. I wanted Australian friends, but somehow learning English on my own as a blind person was just too hard. Despite being comfortable and secure, I was still trapped in my cage of dependency. I told myself that being blind meant I could never be truly free.

All this, however, was about to change: 1985, the year I turned 33, was to be my year of liberation. That year, I found new friends, new learning, and a new life at the RVIB, the Royal Victorian Institute for the Blind. That was the year the horse broke out of the stable!

8
Ben and
the Braille Machine

'Marie, do you know how to read and write?'

'No.'

Lois, the social worker at the Day Centre, must have known that I couldn't read or write, so why was she asking me now?

'Would you like to learn how to?'

The possibility of it went through me like a flash of lightning.

'Yes, please!'

'Alright,' she said. 'You can learn to read and write in braille at the Royal Victorian Institute for the Blind, the RVIB. Just leave it to me and I'll organise everything.'

The following week, Lois came to our home with an interpreter to explain the RVIB to my family and get their permission. Mum was enthusiastic, but Dad was sceptical. 'If she can't see, I don't think there is any way she can learn to read and write,' he said, 'but if she wants to try, she can.'

For a week, all I could think of was the thrilling possibility that I might have my dream of reading and writing after all. I remember the exact day: 12 April 1985. I was ready and waiting when Lois knocked on the door, but I was nervous too. What if I couldn't understand their English? What if I got lost? What if there were stairs everywhere?

We drove for nearly an hour to get to the Institute in St Kilda. As I walked in the door, I felt a strange excitement — as if a whole new world was about to open up, and I had no idea what it would be. Lois led me up some stairs to a room where I was greeted by a man and woman. The man introduced himself as Ben Hewitt, a braille teacher. He said he had impaired vision but could read braille by touch and by sight and could read text by sight. The woman was his student, Jacqui. She said she was studying braille with Ben because she was losing her sight and would soon be blind.

Ben spelled my name out to Jacqui, and asked her to write it in braille so I could feel it. I heard a clanking noise as she typed something on a machine, then they handed me a sheet of paper. I ran my finger over some little bumps that they told me spelled 'Marie Younan' in braille, but the bumps meant nothing to me.

I didn't know English letters and had never heard the alphabet being spoken before. I could not even tell people how to spell my name. Ben said we would start with the alphabet, but I only vaguely understood what that was. I told Ben that it might be too late for me to start learning as I had never been to school. He said, 'Yes, it might be too late, but would you like to try?' I liked him and liked his voice, so I said, 'Yes please!' He said, 'Alright, I'll see you in three weeks for your first lesson.' Later, he told me he could tell by my voice that I was keen to learn — like someone thirsty for a glass of water — and that was why he wanted to teach me.

Three weeks later, on 7 May 1985, I arrived for my first lesson, shaking with excitement. Ben led me to his office and started by telling me that braille was written on a small machine called a Perkins Brailler. He got me to feel his machine, which was like a square metal box, about the size of a shoe box, with six small keys that you pressed with your fingers. Then he showed me how to put thin cardboard pages in and out. The braille machine punched raised lumps onto the pages, arranged in groups. Each group of dots stood for a letter of the alphabet or a number. I was to learn how to read the dots with my fingertips, and learn to write using the braille machine. There were 26 letters in the English alphabet, and I would have to start by memorising the names of the letters and the pattern of dots for each one.

He typed out the first four letters of the alphabet on the machine and got me to feel each group of dots while I said the names of the letters: A, B, C, D. I said each letter and felt the dots over and over again.

After an hour, I started to feel the difference between the groups of dots and began to recognise each pattern. I was ecstatic, and committed myself, from then on, to learn. Somewhere inside me there was a deep determination. The world I came from was stable and safe, but boring. I said to myself that this was my opportunity to take a step out of my small, enclosed world and be in a new kind of world: the world of reading, writing, and the RVIB. I would live in two different worlds and learn to connect the two. My long journey of learning braille through English, and English through braille, had begun.

I immersed myself in the world of braille with Ben as my guide. It was confusing at first, but Ben took it slowly so I could learn three or four letters by heart before going on to the next ones. I felt each of the letters over and over, saying them aloud while trying to memorise the patterns of dots. Slowly, I got the hang of the first four letters. But the names of the next six letters, E to J, kept getting jumbled in my head, and sometimes the groups of dots all felt the same. I was so anxious and embarrassed I wanted to die. But Ben was relaxed and kept on encouraging me. He typed out a sheet of letters divided into smaller groups, and made a tape recording, saying 'First row: A, B, C, D', 'Second row: E, F, G, H, I, J', and so on. When I got home after the first few lessons, I would send myself dizzy trying to remember the letters and what the dots felt like. I had my own little tape recorder, and I sat up in bed at night playing his tape and going over the dots. Gradually, after many, many tries, I learned the names of the letters while my fingertips learned to distinguish the patterns of dots. By July, after three months of hard work, I knew the three main groups that the braille alphabet is divided into: A to J, K to T, and U to Z. I could recite the alphabet, and read each letter with my fingertips while picturing the dots. My fingers and my brain were connecting with each other more and more.

Day after day, I listened to Ben's tapes and ran my fingers over the page. Sometimes I got sick of it, but Ben's kind, relaxed manner made me more confident. I found that if I revised at home what I had learned that day, I was able to remember more next time.

Meanwhile, I was meeting new people who were interested in me and would come over to chat with me. Every day I was welcomed into a friendly community of blind and sighted people in the lounge room or lunchroom. As I relaxed, I talked more to everyone around me and began picking up English by osmosis. The RVIB started to feel like home. Soon I was speaking English without even thinking about it. A small miracle was starting to happen.

For two days a week, from 9.30 until 12.00, I would be at the RVIB. At first, I went by half-price taxi, but the trip from Reservoir to St Kilda Road and back was still very expensive, so Ben organised for Red Cross volunteers to pick me up and take me home. I gave up going to the Coburg Day Centre so I could concentrate all my energy on learning to speak, read, and write in English.

Mum and Dad were happy for me and kept asking me about my braille teacher. Was it a woman or a man? I put off telling them for as long as possible because I thought they would worry if they knew it was a man. Eventually, I had to come clean and tell them. They immediately sent my sister Janet and her husband, Sam, to the RVIB to interview Ben and check whether his intentions were honourable. They arranged a meeting and had a chat about my progress. When they came back, they said, 'Don't worry; he's too old to do any damage!' He was 55 at the time. Nothing more was ever said about it.

Going over and over the groups of dots was hard work. I had never had to concentrate so hard, and for such long periods of time. Ben was always patient and humoured me out of my nervousness about not learning quickly enough or making too many mistakes. Once I had learned the alphabet and the numbers, I knew I would get there. Ben encouraged me to go to basket-weaving and macramé classes for a break from the hard work of learning braille. The craft work was easy and enjoyable. Later, I learned how to knit. With Mum's help, I knitted myself two vests, a blue one and a burgundy one.

Every now and then, Ben would ask me if I could hear the birds singing outside, or he'd get me to feel and name things in the room, such as a vase, or to describe different sizes of paper, and to say whether things were soft, smooth, or rough. Sometimes he would walk me around the garden and teach me to feel and name everything that was in it — the fence, flowers, trees, leaves, bark, the lawn, and the sounds in the street. I never forgot any of the words he taught me, and after six months I was not only reading words in braille but speaking English as if it came to me naturally. As my learning and confidence grew, Ben suggested that I take more lessons, so I started going to the RVIB for three days a week instead of two.

By then I was ready to put words together into short sentences such as 'He is driving a car', or 'She is hungry', or 'This dress is beautiful'. I would arrive home after every lesson with new braille sentences and a new tape recording of Ben reading the sentences, then get to work playing them while running my fingers across the dots. Then I had to learn the abbreviations: words that are shortened to three or four letters in what is called contracted braille. Sometimes I couldn't wait to get home, get into bed, and start listening to the tape. I knew I was doing well, and I wanted to continue experiencing that feeling of achievement.

But underneath I was still plagued by anxiety. My sisters had told me that back in Syria, the teachers would hit them if they made a mistake at school. Maybe Ben would hit me one day if I kept getting things wrong. Every time I made a mistake I apologised profusely, just in case. One day, he asked me why I was so scared of making mistakes, and I told him about my sisters being hit by their teachers in Syria. He picked up a roll of paper and pretended to hit me with it, making a loud noise, saying, 'Now I'm hitting you for all the terrible mistakes you make!', until we were both laughing. 'Please make more mistakes! If you don't make mistakes then you'll know everything, I won't have a job, and they won't pay me. I like your mistakes. We all learn by making mistakes!' My relief was enormous. I learned more quickly and made more progress.

If there were any words I did not know, I would ring one of my nieces and play Ben's recording over the phone, so they could say them in English and translate them into Assyrian. I would make a new recording of my nieces' translations and then play these to myself. I sat up in bed until late, playing the tapes and feeling the sentences until I could understand them, then practised running my fingers across the page more and more rapidly. Sometimes I stayed up until three in the morning, going over the tapes and sheets of braille.

The weeks and months sped by. My store of words kept increasing, and the words found their place in longer and more complex sentences. I was learning how to speak, read, and write in English, all at the same time. Each new word I learned was a small joy. The RVIB became the centre of my life, and, for the first time since arriving in Australia, I was truly happy and never bored.

After a year, Ben said we needed more time, so we worked from 9.30am to 1pm then from 1.30–3pm, which meant I had my own private teacher for five hours a day, three days a week. Day after day, we worked until we were exhausted. Sometimes Ben would lose his voice because he had talked so much, explaining, encouraging, finding new ways for me to see the meanings of words and phrases, and making me laugh. I arrived home dead tired, but always with a small spark of excitement, eager for more.

After two years, I graduated to reading my first book — a children's book called *Pigs and Things*. After that, there were lots more children's books and then adult short stories. Ben would take me to the RVIB library, tell me the names of books, and read a little bit of them to make sure I was interested and that the level was right for me. Then he taught me how to borrow books, and how to order them to be delivered to my home.

One day, he gave me Helen Keller's *The Story of My Life* — a simplified braille version. I was engrossed and amazed by her story. Like me, she was blinded when she was a baby, only she was not just blind, but deaf as well. I cannot imagine what it would be like to have your communication cut off by being both blind and deaf. When she was young, a little girl called Martha, who was the daughter of the family cook, played with her, led her around the garden, and taught her some simple sign language. Martha made me think of my friend Yola taking me by the hand and teaching me things when we were children.

When Helen Keller was six, her parents found a teacher for her called Anne Sullivan, who taught her how to communicate with finger sign language. Anne lived with her as her teacher and close companion for the next 50 years. Eventually, Helen learned braille, and even learned how to understand speech by putting her hand on people's mouths to feel the vibrations. Then she learned to speak by imitating the vibrations that she could feel with her fingers. With Anne Sullivan at her side, Helen Keller became an important writer and public lecturer, famous around the world.

I thought about how much harder it must have been for Helen Keller than for me. Her joy in language was a bit like my joy in learning to read and write in braille. If Helen Keller could do it, then so could I. She showed me that I too could rise above my disability through education and my own determination. And her story made me appreciate how special Ben Hewitt was. Helen Keller had Anne Sullivan as her teacher and friend. I too had a caring and brilliant teacher who taught me how to communicate, taught me about life, and who became my lifelong friend.

Like Helen Keller, I had my own fears and resistances. I had never learned to walk with a cane and was too scared to walk up the stairs at the RVIB on my own. When I arrived, the receptionist would ring Ben to come and lead me to his office. He tried many times to get me to agree to learn to walk with a stick, but I refused point blank. The thought of walking around without a warm, friendly arm to hold onto terrified me. Ben tried everything to persuade me, but I just said, 'No.' His boss, Leanne Thorpe, the manager of the RVIB, was kind and took an interest in me, and she too tried to persuade me to give it a try. They said my life would be better if I was like other blind people and could get around independently. At last I said, 'No! I can't do it! I can only learn one thing at a time. I'm learning braille now. I'll have to stop learning braille if I start learning how to walk with a cane.' Ben just said, 'OK, let's leave it for now and concentrate on braille. You might be ready for it later.'

I also refused for a time his suggestion that I should join classes to learn how to cook and do housework. Yima's voice was still inside my head, telling me not to touch a knife in case I cut myself, and not to go near the stove in case I got burned. Ben said, 'So what if you burn yourself? Sighted people cut themselves or burn themselves all the time; it's no big deal!'

Finally, I went along with some others to learn how to make a cup of tea and a cake. I made the tea using a special tool to measure when the cup was full, so the hot water didn't spill everywhere. When I came to make a cake, my hands were shaking so much that the broken eggs went all over the bench instead of into the bowl. In the end, though, I did it: I mixed the ingredients, put the cake in the oven, took it out with thick oven mitts, and went home proudly carrying a fresh, delicious-smelling cake. The Red Cross volunteer driver that day looked at it and told me it was a 'plain cake'. That was another phrase that I never forgot. Once, I impressed the family by bringing home a tasty lasagne that I had made myself. Secretly, however, I disliked cooking and never got over my fears. Besides, I didn't really have to learn because all the cooking at home was done by Mum or my sisters.

The RVIB trainers taught us how to sweep the floor with a broom, do dusting, and iron clothes. There was a thick plastic strip around the edge of the iron to stop us burning ourselves. We started by ironing a tea towel, then we did pyjamas, then shirts. But I hated ironing. It took ages to lay out each shirt, feel the creases, iron, double check, and then fold each garment. One shirt took me about an hour, and I just didn't have the patience. I have never done any ironing at home because with all my sisters around to do it, I've never had to. But it was another new experience, one that connected me with the world of sighted people and gave me a little more confidence. In the meantime, Mum and Dad were supporting me in everything, and were delighted that I was learning so much.

In 1987, Ben said, 'I'd like to take you to RVIB's holiday camp for blind people for a few days. It's at a place called Romsey, about 90 kilometres north of Melbourne.' I said, 'No, thank you! I'm much too shy, and besides, my parents would never let me go.' A year later, Ben invited me again. This time, he would not hear of me having to get permission from my parents. He said, 'Don't ask them! You're not ten years old! Just say, "Hey Mum, I'm going camping!"'

I did exactly as he said. When I casually told Mum that all my friends at the RVIB were going on the camp, and I was going with them, she said, 'What? How can you?' Then Mum and Dad accepted it, of course, and that was the end of it … another small step towards independence.

Janet helped me pack some clothes, and soon I was in a bus with about 30 other RVIB clients and staff, on my way to a holiday in the country. I was thrilled to be going to a new place away from the city and my family. As I climbed down from the bus, the first thing I noticed was the smell of gum trees and sounds of the bush. Suddenly, I found myself close to nature and far away from anywhere else. The building seemed quite comfortable. I was given the bottom bunk in a room shared with three other women. It was cold outside but warm inside, with a big fire that we would stand around to warm ourselves.

Every day, they took us on a long walk through the forest. I heard bird songs, and smelled bush perfumes and river water. They told us the names of different trees and plants, and got us to touch the tree trunks and leaves. I learned to recognise the songs of magpies, the screech of cockatoos, and the chattering of wrens. My favourite bird was the kookaburra. When I first heard it, I said, 'Where is that terrible loud laugh coming from?' They told me it was the laughing kookaburra. Every time I heard it from then on, I would smile to myself. One day, I heard a banging noise outside, which they said was a kangaroo hopping past the window.

We played games in the evening: dominos, chess, and other games. In those days I could still see a tiny bit of colour, so they gave me blocks which I could use to build things while matching their colours. Sometimes we had discussions about Australia's geography, and Aboriginal history that I'd previously known nothing about. All the time I was learning: about Australia, about how to communicate in English, and how to make friends and be myself in a group.

We had to keep our rooms tidy and make our own beds, which I never had to do at home. Luckily, Connie had taught me, years earlier when I stayed at her home, how to make a bed, making sure to tuck in the sheets and blankets and leave just a little bit of blanket folded under the pillow. I was by now speaking English all the time without even thinking about it. My main friend was a bubbly girl called Ramona Mandy. Ramona worked for some years as a braille teacher, and became well known and respected in the blind community, teaching blind people how to use assistive technology such as talking computers or braille notetakers. Today she lives in Sydney, where she works at the Australian Federation of Disability Organisations.

Relaxing and having fun on my first holiday in Australia gave me a renewed sense of belonging. Being in the bush gave me a special feeling for Australia and what it means to be Australian.

Over the months and years, Ben and I worked hard, laughed a lot, and told each other about our lives. I told him all about my family and my life in Syria, Lebanon, and Greece.

Ben told me that although he was partially sighted, he had attended the school for the blind at the RVIB in St Kilda Road. As a result, he had a special interest in blind people and had many blind friends. During the war, the school was moved to Olinda, in the Dandenong Ranges, where it became a boarding school for blind children. He said he had a wonderful time there, even though the house master was tough and would hit the boys if they disobeyed or were cheeky. One day, three boys ran away, and had caught the train to Melbourne before they were found by police at a train station.

Ben's father had a shoe shop, and after his father died, Ben worked with his mother in a fish-and-chip shop in Dromana, on Victoria's Mornington Peninsula, for many years. After that, he became a teacher of braille and worked in a rehabilitation centre. He was an excellent pianist and organist and played in concerts in the Moorabbin Town Hall.

Ben met his wife Maxene at the RVIB. Maxene was a teacher educator who sustained serious injuries and lost her sight in a car accident, and later became a craft instructor at the RVIB. Shortly after their daughter, Kate, was born, she was diagnosed with breast cancer. Maxene died in 1983, leaving Ben to bring up their then nine-year-old daughter on his own. Maxene's memoir, *The Lion and the Giant of My Dreams* is available as an audiobook in the Vision Australia library.

One day, I admitted to Ben that, at the age of 36, I still had no idea about the facts of life: what happened between married people or even how women became pregnant. It was as if there was a big mystery that everyone in the world except me knew about. I was sick of being kept ignorant of such important matters, as if I was a little child.

Ben explained sexual intercourse to me and how babies are conceived. Then he said, 'I'll book you in to the health-education workshop and they'll tell you everything in more detail.'

As part of the health course, I learned about the heart, the blood, the stomach, and how food is digested. There were life-sized dolls, so I could feel male and female genital organs and learn the names of the different parts. I thought sexual intercourse was a bit shocking, but at least I knew what it was. It was another important step in my belated journey to adulthood. Just because I was blind, I didn't have to be treated like a child and have the facts of life hidden from me.

In some ways, however, my family did still treat me as a child. They loved me and looked after me as best they could, but in their minds, because I was disabled and dependent on them, I was not really an adult. Ben kept on encouraging me to change my relationship with them and be more adult. He would say, 'Don't say "Can I?" You're 36. Just say, "Mum, I'm going to do such and such." Just do it and it will be easier the next time.'

I knew he was right, and began acting more like an adult at home, instead of a well-behaved child. By 1988, Dad was 78 and Mum was 64. They would not be around forever, so I had to be responsible for myself. I also had to separate myself a little bit from my sisters. I was different from them in some important ways, and was learning different skills. I had to be myself, live in my own world, and not try to be like them all the time.

I spent four wonderful years with Ben at the RVIB; four years learning braille, learning English, making friends in my community, and gradually becoming a stronger person. Ben encouraged me to take on new challenges. Sometimes I refused, but mostly he helped me find the courage to try. 'That's OK,' he would say, 'everything is hard for the first time. Why don't you just give it a try and see what happens?'

There were other blind people wanting to learn braille, though, and I couldn't have Ben to myself forever. So, in 1989, Ben prepared me to move on to continue my education in the wider community. 'You need to meet new teachers and find out how sighted people learn to read and write, and learn from them,' he said. 'And they will learn a lot of things from you!'

On my last day as Ben's student, they put on a little party at lunch time, with me as the chef. Sylvia, the occupational therapist, helped me plan the menu, and the RVIB bought the ingredients for lasagne, chicken stuffed with rice and sultanas, and tabbouli, using my mother's recipe. I chopped the parsley, mint, green onions, and coriander under Sylvia's guidance. The lunch was a great success. Everyone was happy and laughing, and I was ready for a new adventure in the wider world, with the RVIB still there as a secure base, and Ben as my dear friend.

9

Learning with Women in a Sighted Classroom

It was my dream to study with sighted students in a proper classroom, and it was also my dread. The old voices were telling me that blind people can't possibly learn with sighted people because they can't read or see what is on the blackboard. But Ben's calm voice was saying, 'You're ready for this, so why not give it a try?'

On my first day, I came by taxi to the Migrant Women's Learning Centre (the MWLC) in Wellington Street, Collingwood. A friendly lady called Veronica came to meet me and escorted me up a flight of stairs into a classroom where other students were gathering. A teacher came to speak to us about the different classes and how they would be organised. But somehow, I couldn't make head nor tail of what she was talking about. Without the printed information on the blackboard or papers being given out, I felt lost, as if I were in a different country. The braille machine sitting on the desk beside me was no help. What was I doing there? I rang Ben that night to tell him it wasn't going to work. He came in the next day and sat next to me in the classroom, telling me what was on the blackboard and explaining the meanings of words. We both realised that I needed an aide to support me and help me negotiate between print and braille. He contacted the Collingwood College of Technical and Further Education (TAFE) to ask them if they could fund an aide to assist me in the classroom.

Then Jill Sanguinetti came into my life, as my teacher in the 'Return to Learning' (RTL) course. The RTL class consisted of about 15 women who had been in Australia for some years, could speak some English, but had never learned English literacy.

Jill was warm and welcoming, and made sure she included me while she was teaching the whole class. She spoke clearly, and I could understand everything she said. I said to myself that, even if I missed out on some things, at least I would be taking in lots of English language and meeting new and interesting people.

Jill began by getting each of us to say something about who we were and where we came from. I was fascinated by the different stories and different accents. Suddenly, I wanted to get to know my classmates better, and I stopped thinking about my own problems. That was the beginning of it. I knew I was in the right place and would stay. When I told them my story of my blindness and how I had waited for many years to come to Australia, they asked lots of questions. I was not the only one who had lived through tough times, or who had problems learning English, and not the only one who felt nervous and inadequate. We were all in this together.

Jill would read out everything she wrote on the blackboard and spell out new words, letter by letter, so I had time to type them into my braille machine. She made sure we understood the meanings of words, explaining them with lots of examples and getting everyone to practise the words in different ways. That way, I came home every day with a list of new words written in braille, and many others in my head that I had picked up from classroom discussions. Each new word opened up my mind a little bit more and gave me another way to express myself in English. Some words I understood immediately from the context; others I struggled with. The first time Jill talked about a 'timetable', I wondered what the connection was between 'time' and 'table'. Was it a kind of clock that somehow sat on the table? I soon cottoned on. It was hard sometimes, but I was learning!

The Collingwood College of TAFE agreed to fund a braille teacher to sit beside me, and that person was Lorraine O'Brien. In no time, she was my friend and personal teacher. With her, my spoken English and braille developed even more quickly. Lorraine loved coming to the MWLC and joining in the learning and the fun of classroom life.

When other students wrote stories, did exercises, or took dictation, I did mine in braille. Lorraine checked the braille before printing the words underneath the dots for Jill to check. Soon the process felt quite normal. I could do nearly everything that the others did, although writing in braille took more time because the keyboard on the machine was a bit stiff and clunky.

It took me a while to get over my shyness. At first, when Jill introduced a discussion or asked questions, I would whisper my answer to Lorraine. She would encourage me to put my hand up and have my say, or else signal to Jill to ask me questions directly. I always guessed when she was signalling because Jill would immediately direct a question to me.

Lorraine took the burden of blindness off my shoulders in many ways, but her warmth and friendship were even more important. We stayed together for four years of study — in TAFE and at the Council of Adult Education (the CAE).

Veronica Wilkes, the MWLC secretary who had guided me on my first day, was my other main friend there. When she offered me her arm for the first time, I could tell that she'd had experience with blind people and asked her about it. She told me that her father had been blinded in a car accident, so that became a small bond between us. Veronica always kept an eye out for me, and often took me upstairs in the morning and downstairs in the afternoon when my taxi came. We became long-lasting friends in the years that followed.

I'll never forget my RTL classmates and teachers of 30 years ago.

There was Chu, a Vietnamese girl who was very friendly and got everyone laughing with her funny comments. There was Vicky, a Greek lady whose husband wouldn't let her come to class, so she had to hide her books and sneak out when he was away at work. Vicky made all her own clothes, and at the end of the year she said she wanted to sew something for each student in our class. She made me a nice flowery summer dress that I loved and wore until it was worn out. There was Nora from the Philippines, who had a very sad life story, but now she was married to an Australian man and happily living in Australia. There was another Vietnamese girl, Phuong, who came to Australia on a boat. When they were at sea, pirates attacked the boat and began stealing jewellery from the women, so she swallowed her ring. We all laughed when she told us how she would check every time she went to the toilet until she found it again. There was Habiba, who said she had left her country riding on a camel. There was Anne from Singapore, whose husband's name was Anthony. They had four children whose names all began with 'A'. And there was Juliette, from Lebanon, who was always singing and dancing in the class. One day, she brought in some music and did a belly dance for us. When Jill described to me how her stomach and breasts were shaking up and down, everyone laughed. They were lovely women from many different cultural backgrounds and with different personalities. We found we had a lot in common when we shared our stories, though.

Jill got us to read books that had been written in simple English especially for adult literacy learners, and Lorraine helped me get audio tapes of the same books from the RVIB library. I remember *I Can Jump Puddles* by Alan Marshall, who was crippled with polio as a baby. He rode everywhere on his pony, and had a happy childhood in the country.

Albert Facey's *A Fortunate Life* also made a big impression on me. He was an orphan who was made to work on a farm, and like me, never went to school. He saw terrible things when he was a soldier at Gallipoli, during the First World War. After the war, he learned to read and write, became a farmer, married, and had a family. After all the hardships of his childhood and his war years, he created a good life for himself. I loved stories about people who were determined to overcome disadvantages, and stories that gave me a sense of Australian people and culture. By then I was feeling more and more Australian, and wanted to belong, not just live on the sidelines as an Assyrian. I thought Albert Facey's story was so important that I made Mum and Dad get the movie version on video. We watched it together while I interpreted for them.

Every day, the students brought food to share, so lunchtimes were like a multicultural feast, with lots of talk about recipes and ingredients. Jill took us on excursions to films, parks, and the Collingwood Children's Farm. The first film I ever went to in my life was *My Left Foot* starring Daniel Day-Lewis. It was about a boy called Christy

Brown, who was born with cerebral palsy and couldn't walk or speak. In the end, he found he could control his left foot, and taught himself to write and to paint with his left foot. It was inspiring to me to see how he overcame his terrible disability and became a useful and loved member of society, a writer and an artist. Of course, I could not see what was on the screen, but with Lorraine sitting beside me and whispering descriptions of what was happening, I could piece it together in my imagination.

Another special teacher was Annie Kelly, who was full of fun and energy. Annie taught us about health and the human body. Whenever she went past, she would tap me two times on the right shoulder. I always knew it was her and could smell her lipstick. Then she would kiss me on the cheek, rub the lipstick off with her handkerchief, and we would both laugh. One day, she gave a lesson about contraception and talked about penises and condoms. I got to feel a condom and blow it up like a balloon. Mum and Dad, even my sisters, would have died if they knew I had been rolling a condom onto a banana as part of my TAFE course. This part of my learning was my little secret.

On International Women's Day, Jill played *I am Woman, Hear Me Roar*, by Helen Reddy. We went through all the words and sang it together. That song was about women being as strong as men and in charge of our own lives. If men try to control us, we will roar like a lion!

Elizabeth Connell was my classroom teacher in the RTL course the following year. She got the students to read a book called *Emma and I* while I read the braille version that Lorraine gave me. It was an inspiring story about a blind girl called Sheila and her relationship with her guide dog, Emma, who took her everywhere and could almost read her mind. In the end, Sheila had an operation and regained her sight. She got married, had a baby, and became a trainer of dogs for disabled people. I don't know why, but I remember the exact moment when we were talking about the book *Emma*, and Elizabeth was explaining the word 'leash'. There was a lovely, warm atmosphere in the room, Lorraine was whispering to me about the leash, and in the exact moment of my understanding of the word 'leash', I felt a wave of happiness. Maybe, in a deep sort of way, I realised that I was letting go of the leash of dependency that had held me back for so many years.

Elizabeth liked to talk about people and relationships, and she explained things in a way that made you want to know more. I used to think she had two voices. She had a special teaching voice that she used in the classroom: a smooth, soft voice like the voice of an angel. Outside of the classroom, she spoke with a normal kind of voice. I did several classes with Elizabeth, including her Technical Orientation Program (TOP) Psychology class, which was a Year 12 subject. In this class I learned about why we behave in certain ways, how childhood experiences affect us, and how our brain works. It was the first time I began to make a connection between my being blind, my family upbringing, and who I was as a person. She explained different theories of psychology, and I took in every word.

One day, the teachers showed us the film *Picnic at Hanging Rock*, about how three schoolgirls and their teacher disappeared when they went to Hanging Rock for a school picnic, almost a century ago. What happened to those girls? Was it just a story, or did it really happen? A week later, MWLC students and teachers got into a bus and drove about an hour and a half to Hanging Rock, where the film was made, and we had our own barbeque–picnic there.

Elizabeth took me for a walk through the bush to explore some of the large rocks and caves. Clinging onto Elizabeth's arm, I stumbled across rough, stony ground covered with grass and bushes. She found a stick for me to hold onto so I could feel where the bushes were. But my stick suddenly disappeared down into the ground. Elizabeth told me I had poked it into an ant hole and there were ants coming up my legs. We couldn't stop giggling after that. I felt some of the tall rocks then we started to go back. After struggling through the bush for about 15 minutes, Elizabeth said 'Oh my God, Marie, I think we're lost.' She started to panic, and I could hear her crying. What if we ended up like the girls and their teacher in the film?

We were calling out to the others, then at last we heard them calling out to us. Everyone cheered when they saw us, and joked that they'd thought we had vanished forever, like the girls in the film. I was exhausted and my legs were all scratched, but I'll never forget the adventure.

One day, I had a scary experience that turned out to be life changing. The MWLC had a flight of stairs at the front entrance, just like at the RVIB. When I arrived every morning, the taxi driver would lead me up the stairs or ring for someone to come down and get me. At the end of the day, someone would lead me down to wait for the taxi. One day, after class had finished and the taxi had been ordered, I waited and waited, but there was no taxi. Everyone had gone home, and I was on my own. I was stuck. I couldn't go back up the stairs safely and couldn't walk anywhere to find someone to help me. In a panic, I slowly made my way back up the stairs, feeling each step as

I went with my feet, certain I would fall down any minute. Luckily, Veronica was still there and called for another taxi, but I was rattled. I said to myself, 'That's it! … It's time for me to face my fears and learn to walk with a cane like other blind people do!' Ben was over the moon when I rang him the next day to tell him I was ready.

It was easier than I expected. An occupational therapist from the RVIB came to the MWLC after classes finished to teach me how to use the cane. I learned to tap it from side to side, check for obstacles in my path, and work out where the stairs were by tapping. It took me several sessions over about a month before I could confidently tap my way along the footpath on my own. On the last day, the occupational therapist made me go downstairs three times, walk along the street, and wait for a taxi. Then she said, 'You've done it, and I have no problems or concerns. I'm out of here!' At last I could walk freely on my own. After clinging to fear and physical dependency for all those years, I had taken another step towards independence.

All the time I was at the MWLC, I had a friend called Janet Younan (a distant relative) who often came to ask me questions and go through the work to make sure I understood everything By 1994, I had done all the available courses, and Lorraine suggested that I go to the CAE to complete a course in Australian history. Twice a week, for three months, we went by tram to study the history of Australia, which I hadn't known anything about before. Again, Lorraine helped me with my braille and helped me find the right audio tapes and braille books. Sometimes we would walk around the shops, or go to Myer and have lunch in a café. For the first time, I got a sense of being in the city, with its crowds of people, and the rumble of trams, and traffic going up and down the streets.

I learned at the MWLC to say what I wanted to say and to be myself amongst Australian friends. I learned that, with support and with opportunities, I could succeed. And I learned that I needed to have both a thick skin and a thin skin: a thick skin to take risks and take the hard knocks, and a thin skin to be sensitive and let the learning come in. I would keep going and never give up the struggle.

10
From Learner
to Teacher

Ben announced his retirement from the RVIB in 1991. A big send-off was planned for such a well-known and loved braille teacher. Leanne said that I was Ben's biggest challenge and his best success story, so I was the one who should make a speech. What an honour! There was much I wanted to say to show my gratitude and respect. Lorraine helped me to write my words in braille, and I practised over and over. When the day came, I stood in front of more than a hundred people and told them what he had given me as a teacher and friend ... and how far I had come in the six years since I'd met him, from a shy, withdrawn young woman who had never been to school and couldn't speak English, to a keen reader and writer with many friends. Ben thanked me and said that I was the one who had done all the hard work.

After I made my farewell speech, a lady called Janet Cronin, who was in charge of fundraising, approached me and said, 'Marie, you are a terrific speaker. You must join the speakers' panel and travel around Victoria with us to talk about the RVIB to help raise funds.' I said, 'No way!' I knew my English language wasn't up to it.

By 1993, though, I was ready. Janet Cronin, Bernadette Jolley, and some of the other blind members of the panel had given me some training in public speaking on behalf of the RVIB. I taped some of their speeches so I could listen to them at home. Then Janet said, 'In two weeks' time, it will be your turn to give a talk to the RVIB Ladies' Auxiliary in a country town.'

My first presentation was to a group in Bacchus Marsh. I sat in the back of the car, numb and nauseated with fear. But I gave my speech. I told them about my childhood in Tel Wardiyat, about my family, how I had been blinded as a baby, how I had not been allowed to go to school or go out of the house, how I came to Australia, and how learning braille had changed my life. When I finished, I knew I had done a good job. A few people were crying. They all thanked me and asked me to come back another time to speak to them. I felt ten feet tall.

After that, we went to a different country town every

month or so to speak to an RVIB auxiliary or groups of school children. One day, I received a mysterious piece of paper in the mail. I showed Ben and asked him what was on it. He said, 'It's your pay cheque.' They were actually paying me to travel around the countryside, meet new people, and speak! The RVIB had not only taught me to speak, read, and write in English, they had also given me my first job.

Speaking to school students was fun. As I went into the classroom, I could hear them whispering about me: 'Here she comes with a stick!' Janet and I would talk to them about blindness, different eye diseases, and how to guide a blind person. I would demonstrate walking with a stick, and show them a talking clock, a cricket ball for the blind that had a little bell inside it, and games such as braille dominoes.

Some of the questions were amusing and others more challenging. Mostly they were questions like:

'How do you know if you are hungry?'

'How do you find your mouth when you are eating?'

'Who puts you to bed?'

'How do you drive your car?'

'How do you mow the lawn?'

'How do you know your own bedroom?'

'How do you tell the difference between shampoo and conditioner when you are having a shower?'

'How do you know the difference between the hot and cold taps?'

'How do you go to the toilet?'

'What does it feel like to be blind?'

I told them that if they closed their eyes, they would still know if they were hungry or not. When they went home, they should get their mother to put a blindfold on them, to see if they can find their mouths with their spoons and forks and eat a whole meal that way.

I would never be able to drive a car, I said, or mow the lawn, but there were lots of other things I could do.

I know my own bedroom because I know where everything is, and because I always burn incense, so it has a special perfume.

I have to put a bit of string or tape on the shampoo bottle, so I can tell the difference between shampoo and conditioner. I know the difference between the hot and cold taps because I know that the hot tap is always on the left, and the cold tap on the right.

I put myself to bed and I go to the toilet the same way as they do, but I have to think more about where I am, remember where everything is, feel my way, and do everything carefully. They should also try going to the toilet with a blindfold on when they were at home, to see what it is like.

I said that being blind just feels normal to anyone who has been blind for a long time. I wish I could see, but I can't. However, life can still be interesting and exciting for people who can't see. They can get married, have children, travel, read books, and have the same sorts of relationships as anyone else.

Ben often asked me about my adventures as a speaker for the RVIB. He said 'One day, you must write your life story. Lots of people will be inspired by it if you do.'

I travelled around schools and other organisations with the panel of RVIB speakers for five years, from 1993 to 2001, telling my childhood story, educating school children and making them laugh. I was also invited to Qantas to do some training with cabin staff about how to lead and work with blind people. Now, I was not just a student, I was a teacher as well: teaching sighted people about the world of blind people, how people live with blindness, and how sighted people can support them.

Deep inside, I was no longer the sad little girl sitting in her corner with nothing to do. I was a different person: a working adult valued and respected by those around me. And I was having the time of my life!

11
My Darling
Mum and Dad

I was flourishing in the midst of study, new relationships and new challenges, all the time relying on my base, the love and support of my family. Mum and Dad had worked hard throughout their years in Syria and Lebanon to provide for the health and well-being of their children. I would thank God, and I thank Australia, that in their retirement they found peace and security surrounded by their son and daughters, grandchildren, and a strong Assyrian community.

At home in Reservoir they were like old friends, talking and laughing in the kitchen. Sometimes Dad would tease Mum by sneaking up on her and giving her a squeeze or a tickle. She would squeal and try to stab him with her knitting needle, then they would have a pretend fight, giggling like little kids.

Dad was a charismatic character, always chatty and good humoured. He liked to be well dressed in smart shirts and well-polished shoes, like a much younger man. My sisters chose his shirts and jumpers carefully when they bought gifts for him, and they always described the colours and stripes to me when they got home from the shops. His favourite colour was light blue. He wore a fresh shirt every day, with a fountain pen in his top pocket. He loved perfumes and had several different after-shave lotions. I could always tell where he was by his after-shave. When we went out together, he would make sure Mum and I looked our best. Mum's shoes always had to be polished. 'Polish your shoes, otherwise I'm not going out with you,' he'd say. 'I like you to look perfect.' He would send me back if my shoes weren't polished or if I had a ladder in my stocking, saying, 'Just because you can't see it doesn't mean you don't have to look good when you go out.' In fact, I was a bit like him, because I too liked to be well-groomed, and I was proud of the smart clothes my sisters bought for me for Christmas or birthday presents.

After I learned braille and began studying, he went from being sceptical that I could learn anything to being proud of my achievements, often boasting about me to his friends. He would say, 'Marie, you can do anything you want — you might even be prime minister of Australia!'

One day in 1989, Dad was working outside in the garden when he fell over and couldn't walk or talk. He was rushed to hospital, where they diagnosed a stroke. After four days, he was home again, and although he slowly regained his speech, he struggled to finish his sentences or say what he wanted. I was the one who could best work out what he was trying to say and would interpret his words for the rest of the family. 'Good on you, Marie,' he'd say. 'You're the only one who understands me.'

By 1990, Mum was 65 and Dad was 79. With no English, they had little contact with the wider Australian community except for shopping and medical appointments. Hanne, Janet, Evette, Sherine, and Antoinette drove them everywhere they needed to go, and we all acted as their interpreters. They were well known in the Assyrian community and had many friends. By then our family had trebled in size and spread in different directions: Mona, Nimo, Rima, and their families were in the USA; Younan, Olga, and their adult children were in the Melbourne suburb of Craigieburn, and Antoinette, Sherine, Janet, Hanne, and Rosa lived near us in Reservoir with their families. Evette, Margaret, and I — the three sisters who remained unmarried — were still living with Mum and Dad.

In 1991, Hanne, her husband Sam, Margaret, and I

put our money together for a deposit so Mum and Dad could buy their first home, a four-bedroom brick home in Massey Avenue, Reservoir. Hanne and Sam moved in with two-year-old Lizzie and baby George, and paid rent to help cover the mortgage. I adored the two little ones and formed a special bond with Lizzie, who today is my housemate, friend, and helper. Hanne, Sam, Lizzie, and George lived with us for four years, while Sam worked in their nut shop in East Keilor.

Soon after we moved into the house, Dad had a second stroke. Once again, he survived and came back to be his usual active self. But three years later, when he was 84, Dad had his third and final stroke. In the morning, he called his hairdresser to come to give him a haircut and a shave. But in the afternoon, he said he felt cold and went to lie down. He called out that his head was exploding, and we knew we had to get him to hospital. I was panicked and kept ringing the wrong number for the ambulance. The paramedics came and took his blood pressure, which was shooting higher and higher.

By the time they got him to hospital, Dad was unconscious, and he never regained consciousness. The doctor said he would not survive the night. All the family crowded into the hospital ward to keep him company and support each other during his final hours. It seemed completely unreal: my lively, funny Dad was leaving us, just like that! He passed away on 14 May 1994, at 11pm.

Dad's good friend, the local priest, put on a special funeral and gave a wonderful eulogy. Even now, Assyrian people sometimes say, 'We remember Nissan, we remember him well.' They talk about how he would always stop to help people get their cars going when he saw them broken down in the street, no matter what time of the day or night it was, and he would never accept anything in return. I missed Dad terribly, especially at our family gatherings. He was a special person and a delightful father. In many ways, he's still with me.

Mum recovered from losing Dad and kept busy with cooking, knitting, crocheting, and sewing patchwork quilts on her sewing machine for everyone's beds, just as she used to do in the old days. In the evenings, everyone would sit and watch TV, while I read books and studied braille.

All the sisters were working. Margaret and Hanne worked at the Nestlé chocolate factory in Campbellfield for about 20 years. They could eat as many chocolates as they wanted at work and buy them cheaply to bring home for the family, so we all put on weight. Sherine, Janet, and Evette worked at Visyboard. Evette was doing hard physical work there in cold, damp conditions. As a result, she became crippled with rheumatism and arthritis, which she never recovered from.

In 2002, when she was 78, Mum started becoming tired and short of breath. I took her to the doctor who ordered a chest X-ray. It was lung cancer and already too late to operate.

After that, my sisters and I took turns to look after her. She went downhill quickly and was soon bedridden. She had several different tablets to take, but I was the only one she would allow to count them out and give them to her. Antoinette would say, 'I just don't know how you aren't confused about which tablets to give her. How do you know the difference between them all?' It was easy, really, because the lid of every container was different, and so I memorised what tablets were in each container. I remembered her dosages, and never got it wrong. I would keep a jug of water and a glass beside her bed. Sometimes I left her pills in a small cup for my sister to give to her, but Mum wouldn't take them until she had double-checked with me that they were the right ones.

Despite morphine, Mum's pain got worse. It was terrible to hear her coughing, moaning, and groaning. I didn't know what to do, or how to make her comfortable.

Sometimes I went into the bathroom, pulled my hair, and cried. Mum never knew she had cancer because the doctors didn't tell her and neither did we. We knew we were living a lie with her but couldn't bear to tell her the truth. She didn't know what was wrong with her, but she did know she was dying.

We asked Mum what she would most like to do while she was still with us. She said her biggest wish was to see her American daughters one more time. Mona and Nimo visited Australia in 2003 to see her, and Rima and her family came in 2004. After Rima left, Mum faded rapidly. Shortly before the end, she said, 'I wish I could give you just one of my eyes so you could see again.'

At that time, I was studying a psychology course at the CAE with the support of a volunteer reader called Chris Wood. But Mum wanted me to be at her side and not leave the house at all, so I had to give up Psychology.

Mum passed away in the Northern Hospital in Epping on 31 August 2004, when she was 80. After she died, I completely lost control. I cried and screamed until the priest told the family to take me away. At the same time, a huge burden had fallen from my shoulders. I thanked God she was at rest and free of pain. Ben sent me a beautiful braille sympathy card.

I couldn't get over my grief at losing Mum. I didn't

want to talk to anyone, and stayed in bed for days on end. When she died, it was as if the centre had gone out of my world. I couldn't even bear to have the radio on, when I was used to listening each and every day. People at the RVIB were worried about me because I was not turning up to any courses or appointments, and they sent a counsellor to talk to me. But it was my sister Sherine and my friend Chris Wood who were the ones who really got me out of the depression. Sherine said, 'Where is your radio? You need to have one on in the kitchen and one on in your bedroom. Turn the radios on, or I promise you, I'll break them!' Then she shouted, 'Bring the radios here, or I'll break them. I'm serious.' That gave me a bit of a shock.

Chris called in several times to see me, too, but I was too depressed to talk to her. Finally, she came around and laid down the law. She said, 'I didn't spend years of my life helping you with your English and your interpreting course, for you to just give up and lie in bed all day! You've got a choice … either get up and get going with your life, or I'm not coming to see you anymore!'

They both jolted me right out of my depression. Mum would not be coming back, and I too would die one day. I should live my life. I didn't want to lose Chris's friendship, so I got up and started going out with her.

After Mum passed, Margaret and I were the only ones

left at Massey Avenue. I was 52 and Margaret was 46. Margaret had never learned to read, write, or speak English fluently. She relied on me for outside communications while I relied on her to do the housework and gardening.

In 2006, when she was 17, my niece Lizzie moved in with us. She was doing a course in Interior Design at the Northern Metropolitan Institute of TAFE at Preston, so it suited her to live with us. Lizzie is marvellous — she helps me with my diary, keeps my email account, and helps me in lots of small ways. Last year she married Hani, an Assyrian refugee who had been living in France. He's working as a brick-layer now, and has moved in with us until they can save enough money to buy their own place.

Mum and Dad are gone, and their remaining children have stepped into their shoes as the next older generation.

12
Becoming
an Interpreter

I love languages and I'm good at them. Over the years, I naturally took on the role of interpreter for Mum and Dad whenever I was needed.

In 1986, when Mum was in the Royal Women's Hospital, there was a Greek lady in the ward who, like Mum, spoke no English. When the nursing staff were struggling to communicate with her, I began interpreting. The nurse said, 'You're a good interpreter. Why don't you do a course so you can interpret professionally?'

Back then, my English wasn't good enough, but the idea stayed with me. In 1997, after 12 years of study at the RVIB, the CAE, and TAFE, I had the English language and the confidence to do it. Ben said, 'You have to give it a go! Why don't you ring RMIT (the Royal Melbourne

Institute of Technology) and ask them about their interpreting course?'

I rang RMIT and spoke to the co-ordinator of the Diploma of Interpreting, explaining that I was blind. She said I would need to come in to speak with Martin, the liaison officer who dealt with disabled students. He was in a wheelchair as the result of an accident he'd had when he was a policeman. Martin was very encouraging and said they could fund a personal reader/note-taker to support me. He also invited me to come to a three-week introductory summer school for would-be interpreting students. The course would consist of several days of intensive language study and other activities at a holiday camp. At the end, the lecturers would judge whether applicants were suitable candidates.

I jumped at the chance. About 20 of us did language work, group work, and different outdoor activities. I even got to fly through the air on a flying fox, which was scary but fun. I made new friends from different language backgrounds, including sign language. A girl called Shirley, who was deaf-mute, befriended me, even though I couldn't see her, and she couldn't hear or speak to me. We communicated through the National Relay Service — a telephone-based service funded by the federal government where relay operators translate information between the spoken word and written text, so that a person who can hear and speak is able to communicate with a person who is deaf or cannot speak.

Shirley was very active, and drove around in a car. She told me about the day a policeman stopped her car, but thought she was pretending when she made signs to him that she was deaf. She had to write on a piece of paper, 'I can't hear or speak,' before he let her go. I lost contact with Shirley after she went to Queensland to open a restaurant.

My other friend was an Egyptian girl called Inez, who was my mate throughout the course, and helped me when I was finding my feet as a new interpreter. Twenty years later, we still chat to each other over the phone.

There weren't enough people for an Assyrian-speaking class, but the Arabic class would qualify me to interpret in my first language as well as in Arabic. At last I got word that I had been accepted.

I went by taxi to RMIT's Swanston Street campus. I went up in the lift, but I had no way of knowing when we were at Level 4 unless I got out and tapped to see if there was carpet in the corridor. If there was no carpet, I had to get back into the lift, and ask people where we were. After I spoke to Martin about it, RMIT installed a device in the lift to announce the levels for me.

My personal note-taker was Fatima, who had just

arrived in Australia from Jordan. She spoke excellent English and worked full time as a computer programmer while attending interpreting classes with me twice a week. Fatima was smart and well-organised, taking notes for me in English and Arabic, and making sure I didn't miss a thing.

The first class was all about confidentiality — how as professional interpreters it is necessary that we keep the identity of our clients confidential, and not talk about them. We would be learning special medical and legal vocabulary for hospital and court interpreting. I had lists of medical vocabulary in Arabic and in English. Any words I didn't know, I would ask my sisters to explain to me or else ring up my GP, who is Egyptian, and ask him what they meant.

One class per week was devoted to practising interpreting. One student would be the client, one would be the interpreter, while the teacher would play the role of the professional, and the rest of the class had to observe and take notes. That way, we all took turns interpreting in front of the class, as well as observing everyone else. The teacher took notes and, at the end, gave feedback regarding clarity, mistakes in either Arabic or English, and any other issues, which we then discussed.

The other class was about spoken English and things

like tone of voice, how and where to sit in an interpreting session, and how to handle emotional situations. For example, if a client was very sick or dying, how to keep a professional distance and protect ourselves emotionally. Fatima took notes of the practice sessions and met me before class each week, and sometimes on Saturdays, to read and discuss the notes with me. That way I could memorise everything I had learned. The teacher taped some of the lectures as well, so I could play these at home.

I threw myself into training for my new career. Sadly, Fatima left at the end of the first year to get married in Saudi Arabia, so I had to begin with a new note-taker, who was terrible. Her English was poor, and her notes completely inadequate. Often, she didn't take notes at all, and when I asked her about it, she would say, 'Just don't worry about it.' She spoke to me rudely, and one day even said, 'Are you crazy?'. I complained to the course co-ordinator, but she said there was nothing they could do. So, I quit, and missed the rest of first semester.

I came back in the second semester with another note-taker they'd found for me, but, again, I was out of luck. This second note-taker was a friend of someone on the course, had no qualifications, and again, did not have the English skills or the interest to do the job properly. I almost quit again but decided to hang in there. Then, at the end of the semester, when we were being tested for our final assessment, she did something quite mad. I was in the middle of being taped as part of the interpreting exam, when she came up to me and started speaking in my ear. I didn't ask her to do this, but the teacher said, 'I can't pass you because she was helping you. Her voice is on the tape.' So, as a result, I failed second semester as well, and had to repeat the whole of second year in 1999. But I learned more by repeating the classes, so it didn't matter.

In the final exam, I had to interpret for someone who had leaves blocking the guttering around their house. I was so nervous that I almost forgot the word 'leaves' and one teacher told me my final mark was 50 per cent, so I might not pass. But two weeks later, I received a letter telling me I *had* passed and was now a qualified interpreter!

I registered with the 'On Call' interpreting agency to be contacted for casual telephone or face-to-face interpreting work.

On 20 January 2000, I received a call from the Royal Children's Hospital for my first telephone job. Could I please interpret for the parents of a baby diagnosed with a hole in the heart? I had to explain to the father what a hole in the heart meant, and that the baby would need to stay in hospital for six weeks for treatment. If the hole didn't close and heal after that, he would need to have an operation. The father was confused and very upset. I had to go over it all several times before he understood. In the end he said, 'Please ask them to do their very best to help my child!' I didn't stop shaking throughout the whole conversation, which lasted about 20 minutes. But I did it, and I got it right!

Inez, my friend from the course, invited me to sit in on some of her interpreting jobs. Our teacher had suggested that after we graduated, we should go to each other's appointments, to observe and learn from each other. Inez was a terrific interpreter; just being able to sit and listen to her work at the Northern Hospital helped my English and Arabic skills and boosted my confidence.

Soon the 'On Call' people were ringing me six or seven times a week for face-to-face or telephone work. Some jobs were straightforward, and others were tricky. The most distressing ones were with people suffering from dementia. There was an elderly woman who was distraught and disoriented after breaking her leg. She was crying out to go home and yelling at the nurses to leave her alone. When she was told she had to stay in hospital, she said, 'How can I have a shower if I stay here? I don't want anyone to give me a shower.' Her words were all mixed up, so it was almost impossible to understand or interpret what she was saying.

There was another lady who seemed quite deranged and didn't have any family members to support her. She pulled at my jacket and my hair, and wouldn't let me go. She begged me to take her with me. When she grabbed my stick, the nurse pressed the button for help. As I went out the door, she was screaming for me to come back and take her with me. I was in a state of shock all day after that.

Interpreting in court was also a challenge. I worked at the Family Court in the city a few times only. I found the conflict too upsetting. I hate to see fighting between husbands and wives, especially when children are involved. Once, I had to go to the Magistrate's Court in Broadmeadows with a couple. We were outside the court waiting to be called in when the man started verbally abusing his wife. Then he said to me, 'Can I borrow your stick, because I want to use it on my wife.' I gave up court interpreting after that.

Interpreting for women giving birth in hospitals was my specialty. On my first birthing job I was on the phone, interpreting for five hours for a woman having a baby in Cairns. I could hear her groaning and screaming, while the midwife and doctor were telling her to push and encouraging her through the contractions. But the baby's head did not come down far enough and it could not be born. I was saying to her, 'It's alright, I'm with you, imagine I'm holding your hand, you'll be alright, you just have to do what the doctors say.' The doctors said they would have to give her a Caesarean, as they had tried everything else. But she would not agree to the Caesar. I had to translate for her why it was necessary, then translate back to the doctors when the woman kept refusing. This went on for hours. Her husband was there, and he said she couldn't have a Caesar because she wouldn't be able to have any more children if she did. This was her fifth baby, and he wanted her to have two more. I had to tell him what the doctor said, that plenty of women have Caesars and go on to have more babies.

About nine o'clock that night, I had to tell them that the child's heartbeat was getting weaker and it would die if she didn't have the operation. Finally, they agreed. I heard the staff talking, and then the baby's cries. It was a boy. They said he was a blue colour, and then they were able to revive him. When I heard he was safe, I felt overwhelmed with joy, relief, and sympathy for the mother. For five hours, I had been at the centre of this traumatic birth, and felt as if I had been right there in the room with them. To me it was a privilege to be part of it and play such an important role.

After that, I assisted in more births and it became easier. I remember one refugee who had only been in Australia a few months. I had to tell her when to breathe in and out, when to relax, and when they were going to give her oxygen. After two hours, the baby came out and started crying. The mother was overjoyed and so was I. When the call was over, I screamed out to Lizzie, 'We had a baby girl!'

Once, I met a lady at our church who said to me, 'I want to thank you. You interpreted for me when both of my babies were born.' Another lady had to be rushed straight to hospital after coming in for a check-up. Shortly after, I received a phone call from the midwife. The mother had asked her to ring me to tell me she had had a baby girl and was fine.

Through this, I also gained some insight into what it is like for mothers having babies when they already have two or three small children. Once, a husband came into the hospital in the middle of the night with two children. His wife said, 'Please tell my husband to take the children and go home. I don't need him here.' Sometimes the midwives ask them whether they want to go on having babies or want help with birth control. Once, a woman said she wanted birth control, but her husband said no, she can't. The midwife said, 'Well, it's not you who has to carry the baby and look after it.'

I love interpreting for the labour ward because it takes me into a special moment in other people's lives. And all my births have ended happily, with a healthy baby in the mother's arms.

13
Farewell but Never Goodbye

At home, I was a traditional Assyrian, living within my extended family and going to church on Sundays. Outside, I was a different person living in a different culture. I had my studies, my braille, and my friendships, especially with Ben.

Ben and I would ring each other up two or three times a week to tell each other what was happening in our lives, and I would ask him his advice on all sorts of things. Within the Assyrian community, there was no way I would think of having a friendship with a man outside of a formal marriage proposal. Ben was a dear friend, but that was all. Our friendship would not have been OK if he was an Assyrian, but as he was an Australian it was never questioned. My family accepted that I was my own person with an Australian life as well as an Assyrian one. And they respected Ben as my teacher.

One evening, he came to have dinner with my family in Reservoir, with me as the interpreter. Mum and Dad liked Ben, and he loved Mum's cooking. We did not meet very often, but our friendship continued to grow over the years. We would meet in the city to go to musicals, sometimes accompanied by his daughter, Kate.

In 2010, Ben turned 80. One day, he rang to tell me the shocking news that he had been diagnosed with oesophageal cancer. Over the next few years, he was treated with chemotherapy, but his condition deteriorated, and in 2012 he was diagnosed with an incurable brain tumour. We continued to ring each other once or twice a week. I always looked forward to our chats and we always had plenty to talk about.

Ben's cancer slowly spread to other parts of his body. By May 2014, he was moved to a nursing home in Toorak, where he spent his final two months. I took a taxi to visit him two or three times a week. He would hold my hand, and we would talk and laugh about the old times at the RVIB. I kept wanting to thank him, and whenever I did, he would say, 'Don't thank me, thank yourself ... you did the hard work. Keep on reading. I don't want you to forget your braille!' He always wanted to hear about how this book was going. 'You must work hard and finish it,' he would say.

Bit by bit, he faded away. Even after he had lost his speech and his sight, he could hear my voice, and he communicated with me by pressing my hand to let me know that he knew I was right there with him. He passed away on 29 June, the day after my final visit. When Kate rang to tell me he was gone, I was overcome with grief. For 30 years, he had been my best and most reliable friend, like an anchor, always wanting to know how I was and always there for me with a kind word and a joke. We had become closer still as I sat with him during his final months.

Ben's funeral was held on 7 July 2014. The chapel was packed with blind and sighted people who had learned from him or known him as a friend or colleague, and there were quite a few guide dogs squeezed in. I sat with Kate in the front row. There were no other family members, apart from a distant cousin. Kate and I were his only family, and she had asked me to give his eulogy.

Kate led me to the front of the chapel to read what I had written in braille. This is what I said:

When I came to Australia, I found it very difficult. I had no education. I knew nothing. I was a little girl in a woman's body. My wish was to learn how to read and write, but I had always been told, *no, you can't, because you can't see*. So I just lived in my own little world. The first day I met Ben was the day my new life started. I went home and said to myself, *I have a big mountain to climb, but I'll give it a try*. After two years, he gave me a book to take home. I was reading to myself in bed when my sister said, 'Marie, are you talking in your sleep?' I said, 'No, I'm reading. My wish has come true.'

Thank you, Ben, for helping me change my life. I used to say to him, 'This is the new Marie, the old Marie has gone.' And now I'm working with refugees, interpreting as a blind woman for my community. Ben, without you I wouldn't be working now. I called myself, 'Lost — Now Found by Benjamin Hewitt.' You helped me to go out into the real world. You brought light into my life. It's not the light you people can see. It's a different light and a different kind of seeing. It's a light that when I read stories of other people's lives, I can understand better what's happening to the people around me. Ben, you will always be part of me. Whenever I read, I say *thank you, Ben*. There is a photo of you and me in my bedroom.

Even if I can't see it, I say good morning to you every morning and I say good night to you. I'm so proud to be part of the big and wonderful legacy that you left behind. You will never be forgotten. You are a wonderful father and you have brought up a beautiful young lady, Kate. She will always be special because of you. My heart goes out to Kate and Ben's many friends for the loss of this incredible man. As difficult as it is today, I know that we will take a piece of Ben's spirit into our lives and hold onto it always.

Many years ago, Ben took me to see *South Pacific*, my first time ever to go to the theatre. He would often sing the songs and we had our favourite songs that we would sing together.

This one is for you, Ben:

'I'm going to wash that man right out of my hair,

I'm going to wash that man right out of my hair,

I'm going to wash that man right out of my hair,

And send him on his way ...'

Farewell but never goodbye, Ben. I will miss you. I thank you always.

14
Working with
Refugee Survivors

When I went to Foundation House, the Victorian Foundation for Survivors of Torture Inc., for the first time, I felt as if I had come home. That was in 2007. I'm proud to belong to the caring, multicultural community at Foundation House, and proud of the work they do for refugees who have survived violence and all sorts of terrible experiences.

Foundation House helps people recover from the trauma of war and political persecution and helps them to put their lives back together in Australia. It has mental health clinics that provide counselling and psychiatric support to clients from refugee backgrounds. There are programs to support families, schools, and regional communities as well as complementary therapies such as massage. Foundation House centres offer services in several parts of Melbourne. I mainly work in the Brunswick centre, which is also the head office, and at the Dallas centre in Broadmeadows. I usually work for two or three days a week, interpreting for psychiatrists, psychologists, and their Arabic- or Assyrian-speaking clients.

Many clients I interpret for are Assyrians who are recent refugees from Iraq and Syria. Almost all the Assyrian communities there been displaced since ISIL invaded in 2014 and Christians were cleared out of Mosul. Thousands were killed and thousands more migrated to different countries, including Australia.

I also meet Assyrians from villages along the Khabur River, in the north east of Syria — villages like Tel Wardiyat, where I was born. The Islamic State of Iraq and the Levant (ISIL) attacked villages and kidnapped hundreds of people, demanding large ransoms from their families. Many of the Assyrian villages in that area are now empty, and churches have been destroyed. Fortunately, all my family members from there have now left. I feel a special bond with Assyrians from my own community who have made it to Australia but are struggling to make decent lives here.

I interpret their stories and hear some of the sad and traumatic things that they have gone through. One woman was sheltering with other Assyrians in a hall when ISIL fighters came in and started killing people. There was a lady there holding the hands of her two small sons, saying, 'Please don't hurt us!', but all three of them died when the fighters threw a hand grenade into the hall. The client who survived that attack was being treated for post-traumatic stress and was taking medication to relieve her depression. After a year of counselling, she was much better and seemed ready to get on with her life. Some clients are strong and manage to recover, but not all of them can.

I feel honoured to hear the refugees' stories firsthand. Often, they are stories that haven't been shared with anyone else. It's important for clients to get their stories out so they can let go of their burden of memory. I hear about things like bombing, imprisonment, physical torture, the loss of loved ones, and stories of life in refugee camps. Often the clients' ability to work or relate to people is affected. Sometimes people are crippled by anxiety, or their relationships break down, or there is domestic abuse or sexual problems. All the stories are different, but they are all sad, and many of them are shocking. I can't help being affected by the stories, even though I have been trained to keep a professional distance. When one client finally got her story out during counselling, she cried a lot and I couldn't help crying with her. At one point, when her story seemed unbearable, I asked for a break so I could take some deep breaths and calm down. We stopped talking and just sat quietly together for a few minutes before continuing the session. The counsellor was very patient and helped her uncover her story, bit by bit. I was glad for her when she finally told us everything. She said, 'Feel for me; I have had this hell in my heart for years, but now I can let it out at last.'

Sometimes people are brought to Foundation House by guards from detention centres in Melbourne. These are the ones who get severely depressed because they have lost all hope of living freely in Australia. Some say life in the detention centre is making them go crazy. They talk about how they want to climb over the wall and be free, or else die. The counsellor tries to calm them down, but sometimes it's impossible. After each session, the guards waiting outside take them back to the detention centre again. It is very upsetting to see people who have escaped war and oppression and come to Australia for a better life only to be locked up when they get here.

The counsellors are very thoughtful, and ask me from time to time if I would like to debrief with another counsellor if the client's story is too distressing, or I feel I might be getting depressed. I always say, 'No thank you, I don't need it.' I can walk out of the counselling room, get a cup of tea or coffee, and leave all the pain and tragedy inside the room. I think that, being blind, I have learned to overcome my own personal sadness and leave it in a special compartment, like saving it onto a computer file. I leave each session behind me so that my mind is clear to interpret for the next session.

Once, a lady was talking about the problems she faced in looking after a blind aunt. When it was over, the counsellor said, 'I'm sorry, but I hope all that talk about her blind aunt didn't upset you.' I said, 'Well, I'm blind, obviously, but hearing the word "blind" and hearing about other blind people doesn't affect me in the least.'

In fact, it's the other way around. Being blind actually has some advantages for an interpreter. Clients have sometimes been humiliated by torture and feel they have lost their dignity. They might feel guilty and ashamed about what happened to them, even though it was not their fault. One man said he didn't want to have a woman in the room hearing his story because he was crying. He said, 'I'm glad you can't see me crying. It's embarrassing.' 'I can hear you,' I said, 'but I can't see you, so you don't have to be embarrassed! I'm here to interpret your words, not to judge you.' He was alright after that.

After each session, the clients always thank the counsellor and they thank me. One man said, 'I thank you, and I thank Foundation House from the bottom of my heart! I hope God brings you a beautiful house! I was anxious, but you made me feel relaxed. Your speech is very clear, so now I understand everything!' I said, 'Well, it's my job, and it's my responsibility to give the right message in each language.'

I am learning all the time from counsellors who know how to bring out people's stories, how to hold their experiences and give them emotional support. I witness the clients' pain and express it for them as I translate their words into English. Hearing me repeat their stories in English is part of the process. I think that when clients tell stories in their own languages and hear them translated into English, and the counsellors' English language responses are translated back to them, something important is happening. It is as if by reaching across the language and cultural barrier, Australian society is showing that it cares about them and their trauma. The clients' pain is taken in, acknowledged, and respected in two languages. This is how the clients' grief can be reduced bit by bit, and traumatic memories soften and become manageable, so the memories don't overwhelm their lives. When they are given professional support and advice in their own language, it means they don't have to feel anxious about missing something, or struggle to understand every word.

They can relax more, and take in the suggestions and feedback that are offered to them.

I have seen distressed and traumatised people dealing with their past suffering bit by bit. After a year or two of counselling, they go out and get on with their lives with a stronger sense of themselves and hope for the future.

I have realised how lucky I am. I might be blind, but I have never been tortured or locked up, and I don't suffer from depression or suicidal thoughts, like some of our clients do. Before, I used to say to myself, 'I wish I had lost a leg instead of my sight,' but now I say, 'Thank goodness I'm only blind. I haven't been tortured, and I'm lucky to be able to help these people by interpreting for them.'

My heart goes out to clients who carry so much pain inside them. I think of Yima as a young woman in her 20s, holding Dad's hand and the hand of her little cousin, as they walked for days along a rough mountain road in freezing weather. I think of her looking through the window of the women's prison and seeing dead bodies. I think of Sarah and all the babies she lost, and the pain in her feet that she could still feel 50 years later. I think of Sam, always jovial and joking, never talking about what *he* must have gone through. They survived the death march, walking through the harsh landscape, desperately trying to keep themselves and their children alive.

I wish my parents and grandparents could have had counsellors like the ones at Foundation House, to help them talk about their pain. Now I respect them even more for the loving care they gave to us after experiencing such great suffering. Their stories live on inside me and make me want to do the best I can for the clients I work with, and for my community.

15
If Only We
Had Known ...

As a child, I was traumatised by being blind: locked out of play, school, and social gatherings; locked into dependency, boredom, and a thousand small frustrations. Thanks to Australia, and thanks to more people than I can name, I have moved far beyond the enclosed world of my childhood and into a world of relationships, work, and personal freedom.

Speaking four languages, I can move easily between four different cultures. Like other disabled people, I have come to terms with my disability and often forget about it altogether.

The grief of being blind has faded, but underneath there was another grief. For years, I agonised over my poor grandmother blinding me with cochineal. I would go over and over it in my mind, about how she must have felt, having injured an innocent baby, her granddaughter, in such a terrible way. I would lie awake at night pitying her for her self-blame as I imagined it. I felt guilty about her guilt. And there was a lingering mystery: what really made me go blind? Was it Yima and the cochineal, or was it something else?

Last year, Jill did some research and found out about 'congenital' or 'infantile' glaucoma. I was amazed. No-one had ever told me that people can be born with glaucoma. Since then, I have learned that infantile glaucoma is caused by a birth defect that affects about one in 10,000 babies. As a result of the defect, fluid cannot drain out of the eyeballs properly. The fluid becomes trapped, building up pressure within the eyes. The pressure damages the optic nerve and leads to blindness if it is not treated. Symptoms of infantile glaucoma include swollen, teary eyes, and aversion to light, although these symptoms may not appear until the baby is several months old.

Until I heard about infantile glaucoma, I believed the family story that it was the cochineal eyedrops that had made me go blind. But then I began to question it. What if the eye infection I had when I was six months old was in fact infantile glaucoma? What if the eye medicine the American doctor had given me, shortly before he died, was for glaucoma?

When I went to Chicago, I met an elderly lady, a family friend called Emily who remembered me as a baby in Tel Wardiyat. Emily was the one who had suggested that Mum should take me to the American doctor who was going around villages in 1952 to help people with eye problems. She said to me, 'I remember what your eyes were like before the doctor came. Oh, you poor little darling! I can see you right now, being held in your mother's arms. Your eyes looked terrible. You could hardly open them, and they were streaming with tears.'

I now know that closed, streaming eyes are symptoms of infantile glaucoma. So that must have been the disease I had then, rather than an ordinary infection. Did the glaucoma cause my blindness, or was it the cochineal? Glaucoma damages the optic nerve but does not scar the corneas. But my corneas had gone white in just 24 hours, blocking out the light. The glaucoma could not have done that.

According to the medical literature, corneas can be harmed by coming into contact with different substances. The red dye in cochineal comes from crushed insects and is preserved in an acidic solution that could harm the skin, eyes, or respiratory tract. So, it is highly likely that acidic cochineal drops, bandaged into the eyes of a small baby for 24 hours, could have damaged her corneas.

My corneas were opaque, otherwise they would not have attempted corneal transplants in the hope of restoring my eyesight. So, the only conclusion is that after being born with congenital glaucoma, my eyes were damaged for a second time by Yima's cochineal.

So now I know! My poor baby eyes suffered a double whammy — first from infantile glaucoma and then from the cochineal.

If it hadn't been for the glaucoma, my corneal transplant operations would probably have been successful, as they are in 90 per cent of cases, and my sight would have been restored 30 years ago. But the transplanted corneas would have been rejected because of the pressure in my eyeballs, which had been caused by the glaucoma.

My grandmother made a mistake, but her mistake would have been fixed by the corneal transplant if it weren't for the pre-existing glaucoma, which after so many years had become incurable.

Oh Yima, if only we had known!

16
Yesterday and Today

Australia has been my home for 42 years now. I'm well settled with family, work, my Assyrian community, and some excellent friends.

One of these is Veronica Wilkes, my friend at the MWLC. In the early 90s, she invited me to her home for dinner and to meet her husband, Richard, and two small children. I was shy at first, but with Veronica's warmth and sense of humour, I was soon laughing with them and enjoying myself. After they moved to Bairnsdale, a town in Victoria's East Gippsland region, they invited me to come down and spend a weekend with them there.

Janet's husband, Sam, was to come with me on the train to the nearby town of Sale, where Veronica and Richard would meet us on the station. Sam was thrilled to accompany me, as he had never been on a train in Australia before. However, he did not know there were toilets on the trains, and when the train stopped along the way, he got off to look for a toilet. But the train went after a few minutes, leaving him stranded at Traralgon and me on the train on my own. I turned up at Sale without him, while he had to wait four hours for the next train. We had a good laugh when we finally picked him up at Sale station. Veronica and Richard treated us like royalty and drove us around different tourist places in the countryside. Veronica described all the details of hills, the trees, the paddocks, the farm animals, the small towns, lakes, and forests, so I could see everything in my mind's eye.

I visited them in Bairnsdale several more times. Once, when he was small, my nephew George came with me. They took a great interest in him and he loved them. Veronica would visit me at Massey Avenue when they came to Melbourne. Her family opened their hearts to me and my family, and in 2009, they invited me to come to Bairnsdale for the wedding of their daughter, Catherine. I had known Catherine since she was five or six, and she had grown up to become a beautiful ballet dancer and teacher of ballet. I was thrilled to be at their family wedding, accompanied by my niece Christina.

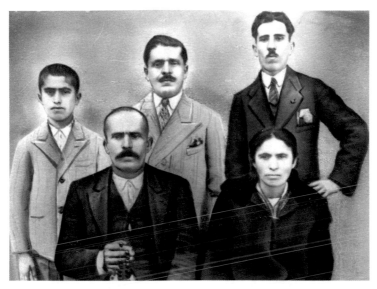

Yima (Christina) and her husband, Gando, with Dad (top left) and two uncles when they were living in Greece, c.1923.

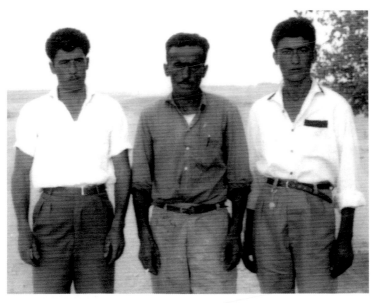

Dad with Michel on the left and Younan on the right, c.1964.

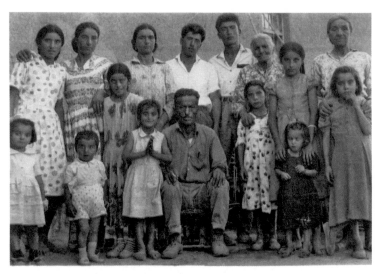

My family outside our home in Tel Wardiyat, c.1962.
From top left: Nimo, Antoinette, Samira (Mum), Michel, Younan, Yima (Dad's mum), Janet, Sarah (Mum's mum). **Bottom left:** Esther (Antoinette's daughter), George (Antoinette's son), Marie (me), Shamiran (Antoinette's daughter), Nissan (Dad), Evette, Rima, and Mona. (Sherine and Margaret are missing from this family portrait.)

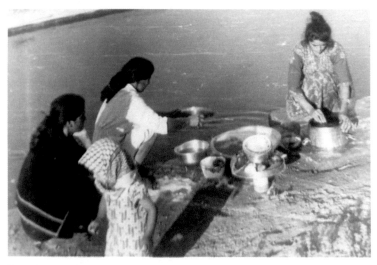

The Younan sisters washing dishes in the canal at Tel Wardiyat, c.1968.

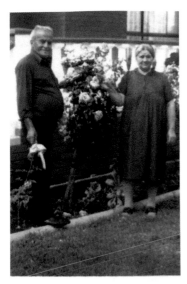

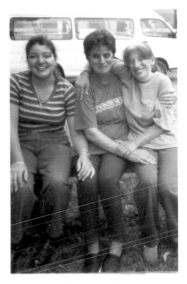

Dad and Mum in the rose garden at Leech Street, *c.*1987.

A happy day with friends from the Coburg Day Centre.

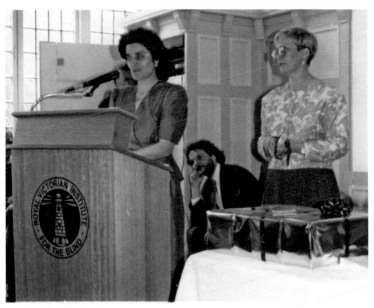

Me making my speech to Ben at his RVIB farewell in 1991.

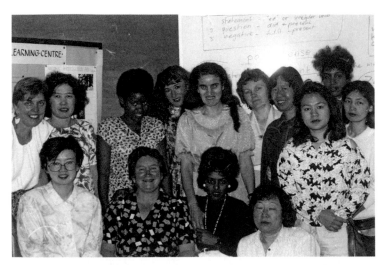

The Return to Learning Class. Jill Sanguinetti is on the left, and I am in the middle.

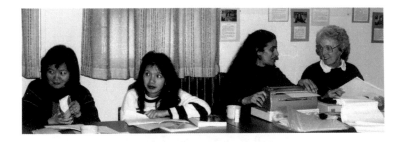

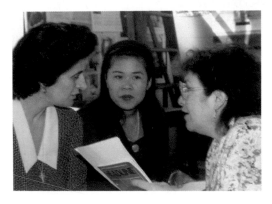

Above:
With my braille aide, Lorraine O'Brien, and MWLC students.

Left:
Conversation with student friends.

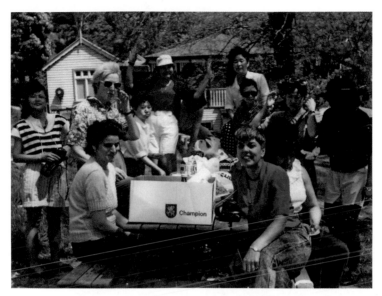

Picnic at Hanging Rock. I am on the left at the front and Jill is on the right.

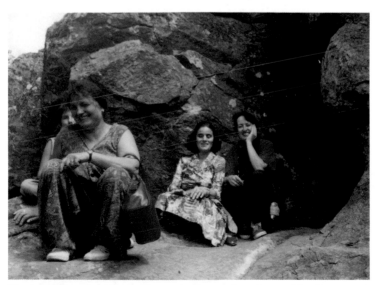

Picnic at Hanging Rock. Elizabeth Connell and me with other MWLC students.

Me on a flying fox at the RMIT camp for students joining the Diploma of Interpreting course in 1998.

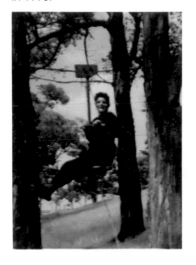

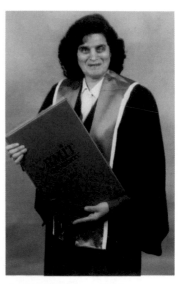

Graduating from RMIT with my diploma in 1999.

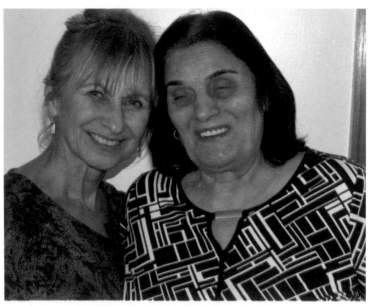

With my friend and helper Chris Wood.

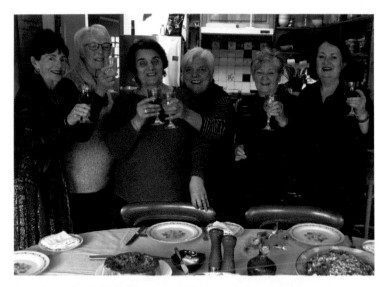

Reunion with MWLC friends in 2018. **From left:** Annie Kelly, Lorraine O'Brien, me, Jill, Veronica Wilks, and Elizabeth Connell.

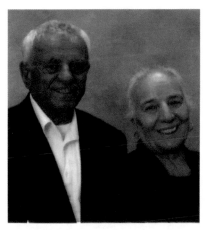

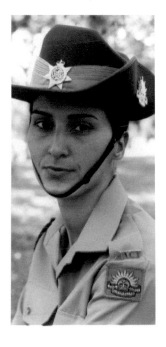

Above:
My eldest sister, Antoinette, with her husband, Peter.

Right:
My niece Elizabeth (daughter of Michel and Rosa).

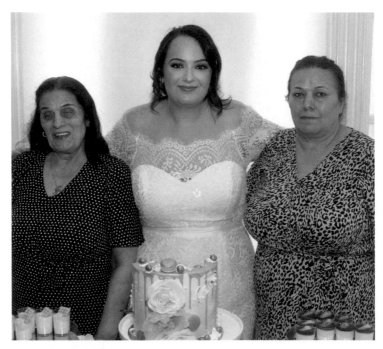

With my niece Lizzie and sister Margaret at Lizzie's wedding shower.

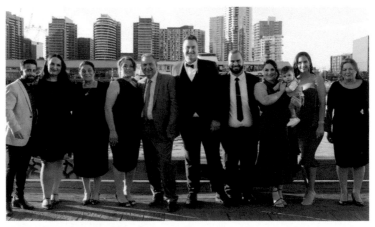

Family party. **From left:** Hani (Lizzie's husband), Lizzie, me, my sister Hanne, brother-in-law Sam, nephew Joseph, nephew George, his wife, Souad, holding baby Samuel, my niece Christina, and my sister Margaret.

Fifteen years later, when George got married, he invited Veronica and all her family to his wedding as guests of honour. His bride, Souad, was Lebanese, and they put on a huge wedding party for more than 300 guests. There was Western, Assyrian, and Arabic music, and speeches made in three languages. Again, Veronica sat next to me, describing everything that was going on. They were delighted to be part of such a grand multicultural wedding, and said it was one of the best things they had ever done. Going to each other's weddings sealed the lifelong friendship between our two families.

Another great friend is Chris Wood, who came into my life in 1996 as a volunteer with the RVIB. At the time she was a real estate agent and mother of two young children, but she wanted to do something to help blind people. She was sent to me as a reader and note-taker so I could do the Victorian Certificate of English (VCE) Year 11 English correspondence course. Chris helped me to enrol, and we did the whole course together. The RVIB sent me talking books or braille versions of the books on the curriculum. Chris read out the guidelines and assignment tasks, and we talked about the books, the ideas, and each of the assignments. Then I would tell her what I wanted to write in the essays and assignments. Chris would take notes and put my ideas into written form, which we would then go over together. We met for several hours once a week at her home or my home, and talked a lot on the phone. Mum and Margaret would make tea and coffee for us, and Chris also helped them with all sorts of paperwork they had to deal with. After that, she helped me with my CAE Psychology class before I had to leave that to look after Mum. She came to our home so many times that she became like one of the family. Chris was good fun. We told each other what was happening in our lives, including things that I couldn't talk about with my sisters. As I described earlier, her friendship got me through my depression after Mum died. These days she often rings me, and we always have lots to talk about.

I have kept in touch with Lorraine, my braille classroom aide in the early 90s, and from time to time go to reunions with Jill, Annie, Elizabeth, and other MWLC teachers.

A few years ago, I invited Jill and Elizabeth to an exhibition of 'The Wonders of Ancient Mesopotamia' at the Melbourne Museum, so I could share that history with them. I'm proud of the ancient history of my Assyrian forebears, although I grew up knowing little about it. Nearly everyone in the Assyrian community went to see it and everyone was talking about it.

We learned about the ancient Assyrians who built a mighty civilisation and ruled for more than 1,000 years, from about 2000 BC to 600 BC. That was in the Bronze Age, when agriculture and writing first developed and the first large cities were built. The three of us were engrossed for over an hour. Jill and Elizabeth described the objects displayed and read out the information about each one. I pictured in my mind the carvings, the pottery, the gold jewellery, and the 3,000-year-old tablets inscribed with early Aramaic writing. When we got to the Babylonian Gates of Ishtar, I was able to feel the display model, which had a carving of a winged lion with a human head on it. We learned that the winged lion represents Ishtar, the goddess of fertility, love, and war. Today, it is known as a symbol of Assyrian and ancient Mesopotamian culture.

In the museum shop there were some earthenware urns that I could lean down and feel. Oh my God! Those urns were just like the urns Yima had used for storing wine in her shed at Tel Wardiyat!

After losing my sight completely during the 80s, I was plagued by recurring infections in both of my eyes. The pain felt like being stabbed in the eyes with a knife. My eye doctor said that there was no point in trying another transplant, and that the only way to stop the infections was to have my eyes taken out and have glass eyes put in.

'I'm scared,' I said to Ben. He said, 'Glass eyes will make you happier and free of pain.' He introduced me to Kay Hancock, a telephonist who had glass eyes. We met for a coffee, and she took her eyes out so I could feel them and feel how each eye was marked for left or right. She said I would have to take them out and wash them every two weeks, and leave them in a glass of special liquid overnight. She said she felt fine with her glass eyes, so I knew I would be OK as well.

They took my first eye out in 2001, and six weeks later they put in a clear glass eye to keep the eye socket open. In 2006, I got my second glass eye. Now I'm very happy with my glass eyes. Every two weeks I leave them in the bathroom soaking in a glass. I say to people, 'Be careful of my eyes in the bathroom!', or, 'Would you please keep an eye on my eyes!' Everyone in the family takes an interest in my glass eyes. One day, Lizzie and I were together when I scratched my eye and my glass eye popped out onto the floor. She found it for me while we both giggled. Later, my nephew George bought me fancy reading glasses to give me a different image.

Many blind people have guide dogs, but I've never had the confidence to care for a dog or trust a dog to keep me safe from traffic. Blind people regularly take public transport using dogs or just their canes to help them get on and off and find their way around. I'm too anxious to take public transport on my own. Instead, I take half-price taxis anywhere I need to go, and rely on them for travelling to and from my interpreting appointments. I know the women on the switchboard at SilverTop, and my favourite drivers usually take the job when they know it's me.

Taxi drivers usually come to the door, guide me to their taxis, then guide me to the door when we arrive. The only problem I've had has been with drivers who, because of their religious beliefs, aren't supposed to touch women apart from wives and family members, so they won't guide me to and from the car. This has led to a few funny incidents. One day, a driver tried to take my arm with two fingers instead of offering me his arm. I said, 'I'm not going to bite you, let me take your arm.' But he didn't, and as I was coming down the steps he stood with his back to the wall. I got confused and lost my step, twisted my ankle, fell onto my knees, and ended up with my head poking between his legs. He was yelling 'No! No! No!' as if I was attacking him. He wouldn't lift me up, I think because he was holding onto his trousers for dear life. I was stuck on my knees with my head in his crotch and couldn't move. Janet and Margaret came running out to see what was going on. 'What are you doing down there?' they said. I replied, 'I'm looking for gold!' After they helped me up, the driver ran to his cab and drove off, while the three of us laughed our heads off.

Being blind is a constant struggle, but of course, sighted people also have difficulties that they struggle with. Today, my life is filled with more joy than sadness … much more!

There have been long gaps in writing this book when work, illness, and death have taken over. In 2015, there was a big influx of Assyrian refugees, and I was called on to interpret almost every day. Interpreting is very tiring, as you have to concentrate 100 per cent to make sure you hear every word and get every detail right. After three or four hours in a row, I've had it. On weekends I slept and went to the usual family dinners and gatherings. That year, we made very little progress with our book.

In February 2017, my younger sister Evette died suddenly in her sleep. She was only 59, a diabetic, but not critically ill. The autopsy revealed no clear reason for her death. The doctors thought that the drugs she was given for arthritis and rheumatism caused her diabetes, and they may have caused her early death. But suddenly she was gone.

Dear Evette, I admired you so much for your independent spirit, your physical strength, and the row of tennis trophies that you kept on your mantlepiece!

I couldn't work on my book for six months until I recovered from the devastation of losing Evette. I used to enjoy saying 'we are ten sisters.' Saying 'we are nine sisters' sounds a little bit sad in comparison.

Then I was laid low with a serious illness for most of 2018. But, thanks to the wonderful medical treatment I received, I made a full recovery last year and am back to my old self.

Assyrian communities in Australia are held together by our churches and our Assyrian-language radio programs. Hanne and I go to St Abdisho's Assyrian Catholic Church in the northern Melbourne suburb of Coolaroo. It's the centre of our community and is often packed with 800 or more people. Although it's a Catholic church, the prayers and rituals are nearly the same as those in the Assyrian Orthodox and Protestant churches. The main difference between our church and the Orthodox church is that we Catholics celebrate Easter and Christmas on the same dates as mainstream churches do, instead of when the Orthodox Russian and Greek churches do.

Most people in the congregation have never learned to read Assyrian script so they cannot read the prayers or scriptures that are passed around on cards. Instead, the priest chants the prayers and psalms, and the congregation chants in response. When hundreds of people are chanting prayers in unison, I feel a deep connection with the church and my community. I love the singing of the women's choir as the choristers walk down from the choir stalls to the front of the church for Holy Communion. Everyone lines up to receive a wafer of bread and sip of wine from the goblet held by the priest. It usually takes over an hour as the deacons direct the congregation to come forward from the pews, line by line, to receive communion and be blessed by the priest.

At the end of the service, ladies stand at the front of the church to offer everyone a gift of food as they leave the church — often it is warm dolma wrapped in pita bread.

Nowadays, the young people — children of the third generation — speak and understand very little Assyrian. They go to Sunday school to learn about our language and culture, but most of the time the youngsters are more Aussie than Assyrian in the way they speak. Now, the community is trying to raise funds for an Assyrian high school in Melbourne, so our young people will learn to speak Assyrian and be part of preserving our language and culture.

On Sunday afternoons, from 4–5pm, I tune in to Melbourne's Radio 3ZZZ for the Assyrian language program, 'Voice of Assyria', broadcast by Jacob Haweil. Jacob is chairman of the Australian Assyrian Arts and Literature Foundation and works with me as an interpreter at Foundation House and elsewhere. The program broadcasts news, songs, poems, historical stories, and interviews to Melbourne's population of more than 13,000 Assyrians. It helps keep our community connected and our national heritage alive. I also listen to Vision Australia Radio, which broadcasts readings from newspapers and magazines, as well as some specialist programming of particular interest to the blind and low-vision community.

There are now more Assyrians living in Western countries than in our homelands in the Middle East. Today, I call myself an Assyrian-Australian. I'm proud of both parts of my national heritage.

The Younan family of Tel Wardiyat has now grown into a tribe of more than a hundred. My brothers and sisters have given me 27 nieces and nephews, most of whom have found partners, settled down, and had children of their own. At last count, I had 28 great-nieces and -nephews, with more babies on the way.

Auntie Yonia from Ras al Ain and five of her children live in Germany. Other relatives went to the Assyrian community in Chicago. I have five first cousins in Melbourne, six in Germany, three in Canada, and one in New Zealand: fifteen first cousins all together. We're also in touch with second cousins who live in Athens and elsewhere around the world.

My nieces and nephews have taken different pathways: there are shopkeepers, business people, carpenters, builders, clerical workers, a lawyer, a university administrator, a hospital secretary, a nurse, a psychologist, and one niece is in the Australian Defence Force. Most have married Assyrians and are active in our community.

Long ago, I was never invited to weddings, parties, or other celebrations. That has changed completely. Now I am welcomed to all the parties and get-togethers. I love the conversations, the atmosphere, the music, and just catching up with friends and families.

Last year, my nephew George and his wife, Souad, called a big party after they had learned the sex of their unborn child. The announcement was to be made in a dramatic way. Instead of simply telling everyone the sex of the baby, they hung a large balloon from the ceiling, filled with small bits of paper. When George and Souad burst the balloon, a cascade of paper would tumble out.

If the baby was to be a boy, the shower of paper would be blue; if it was to be a girl, the shower would be pink. At a given moment, George and Souad popped the balloon together with a needle. Everyone clapped and cheered except me. How could I, when I couldn't see the balloon or the colours? Souad's mum put her arm around me and told me that the papers were blue. Suddenly, I burst into tears: tears of happiness for them and sadness that I had missed out on that special moment. Souad hugged me and started crying too.

Their baby, Samuel, was baptised recently in a ceremony in St Abdisho's church, and a large celebration was held in the reception centre next door.

Long ago, I was too scared to hold babies in case I dropped them — and because not being able to see them made me feel sad. Not anymore. Samuel is now a bouncing nine months old. Last week, I cuddled and danced him on my lap while he laughed and squealed with joy. When I went to stop, he flapped his little arms up and down to make me keep going.

He will always be part of my life and I will always be part of his.

Background Notes

Ancient Assyria

Assyrians trace their lineage back to 2500 BC, when Assyrian kings ruled the city-state of Assur in ancient Mesopotamia. The early Assyrians developed an agricultural economy and built large, fortified cities near the Tigris River.

By around 900 BC, the Assyrian kings had increased their territories and formed a powerful military empire known by historians as the Neo-Assyrian Empire. The Neo-Assyrians united most of the present-day Middle East by military conquest. Their lands stretched from the Tigris and Euphrates across the territories of modern-day Iraq, Israel, north-eastern Syria, south-eastern Turkey, and north-western Iran. According to some historians, the Neo-Assyrians formed the first real empire in history: they forged weapons out of iron and employed sophisticated military tactics. In 631 BC, the empire began to disintegrate following civil wars and attacks from the Persians, Babylonians, and Chaldeans.

Archaeological sites at Nineveh, Assur, and Nimrud contain evidence of the Neo-Assyrian empire. Assyrian sculptures and artefacts found at Nineveh, near the Iraqi city of Mosul, can be seen in museums around the world. The Islamic State of Iraq and the Levant (ISIL) occupied the site during the mid-2010s, during which time they bulldozed many ancient monuments before Mosul was recaptured by Iraqi forces in 2017.

Christianity became established amongst Assyrians as early as the 1st century AD. Assyria dissolved as a geo-political entity after the Arab-Islamic conquest of around 700 AD. The Assyrian people have survived as a people and have preserved their heritage as an ethnic, linguistic, and religious minority in the Middle East despite centuries of persecution.

The Aramaic languages

Ancient Aramaic arose as a Semitic language spoken in the region of Palestine and the Tigris River from around the 10th century BC. During the Neo-Assyrian Empire it spread throughout most of Mesopotamia until it was replaced by Arabic in about 650 AD. Hebrew and Assyrian developed from ancient Aramaic, along with a number of related Aramaic languages still spoken in scattered communities in the Middle East.

Today, Assyrian Neo-Aramaic (or Syriac) writing is used mainly in religious and historical texts. The main speakers of Neo-Aramaic are ethnic Assyrians who speak either Assyrian Neo-Aramaic or Chaldean Aramaic. Both of these dialects are spoken within Assyrian communities in Australia.

The Australian Assyrian Arts and Literature Foundation (AAALF) has a Syriac printing press that it uses to produce historical and cultural works that preserve and promote the history, language, arts, and culture of Assyrian people living in the diaspora. Assyrian language and writing are taught to children by priests and deacons of the church at Sunday schools. An Assyrian high school has been established in Sydney to teach young people and keep Assyrian culture and language alive. Melbourne's

Assyrian community are also planning to establish an Assyrian high school in the next few years.

The Christian genocide

The oppression of Christians goes back to the 1st century AD, when members of the small Jewish sect proclaiming Jesus as the Messiah were persecuted by both Jews and Romans.

Throughout the 16th, 17th, 18th, and 19th centuries, the ruling Ottoman Empire subjected Christian communities to waves of expulsion, forced Islamisation, and massacres, especially in Albania, Bosnia, Bulgaria, Kosova, and in northern Greece.

Between 1843 and 1847, the massacre of Badr Khan in the Hakkari region of Turkey resulted in the slaughter of more than 10,000 Assyrians, and thousands more were sold into slavery. In the Hamidian massacres of 1894–1896, an estimated 80,000 to 300,000 Armenians and Assyrians were killed in anti-Christian pogroms. The Adana massacre in 1909 resulted in the deaths of a further 30,000 Armenians and 1,500 Assyrians.

Between 1915 and 1921, the government of the collapsing Ottoman Empire (the 'Young Turks') carried out mass killings of Eastern Christian populations in Anatolia, Persia, Northern Mesopotamia, and The Levant, resulting in an estimated 3.4 million deaths: 1.5 million Armenians, 750,000 million Assyrians, 900,000 million Greeks, and 250,000 Maronite Christians. Indigenous Christian populations who had existed in the region for thousands of years were decimated.

Historian David Gaunt has written that the Assyrians of the Hakkari area, where Marie's four grandparents came from, were targeted in a full-scale ethnic cleansing during the First World War. Homes were burned, property destroyed, and women were forced into sexual slavery. It was reported that in one district of Hakkari, only 17 Assyrians survived attacks on 41 villages.

During the First World War, when the Ottomans and Germans were fighting against the British and the Russians, Assyrians were caught up in a web of imperial power struggles. The British recruited Assyrians to fight with them against the Ottomans and Germans. But when the Russians withdrew in 1917, the British failed to protect the Assyrians and thousands were slaughtered. The Germans encouraged their Ottoman allies to declare a jihad against the Christians, who were allies of the British.

The United Nations has yet to formally recognise the Christian genocide, despite formal recognition by 32 governments around the world.

The genocide of 3.4 million Assyrian, Armenian, and Greek Christians was formally recognised by the United States in a resolution adopted by the House of Representatives in October 2019.

For further information on the Christian genocide, see:

Travis, Hannibal (2006) '"Native Christians Massacred": The Ottoman Genocide of the Assyrians during World War I.' *Genocide Studies and Prevention: An International Journal*: Vol. 1: Iss. 3: Article 8. Available at: https://scholarcommons.usf.edu/gsp/vol1/iss3/8

Gaunt, David, 'The Ottoman Treatment of Assyrians', in Grigor Suny, Ronald; Muge Gogek, Fatma; Naimark, Norman M., (eds.) (2011). *A Question of Genocide: Armenians and Turks at the End of the Ottoman Empire.* Oxford University Press.

Shirinian, George (ed.) (2017) *Genocide in the Ottoman Empire — Armenians, Assyrians and Greeks, 1913–1923*, Berghahn Books, New York.

The Assyrian diaspora

The Assyrian homelands include parts of present-day northern Iraq, south-eastern Turkey, north-western Iran and north-eastern Syria. However, following the Ottoman genocide, the Simele massacre in Iraq, and the Lebanese civil war, hundreds of thousands of Assyrians have migrated from the Middle East and established Assyrian communities in other parts of the world. In the last 20 years, the persecution of Assyrians by Saddam Hussein and other Ba'athist regimes, civil wars, and attacks by ISIL have forced thousands more to flee from their homelands.

The total population of Assyrians worldwide was estimated by the United Nations High Commissioner for Refugees in 2015 to be 2 million people. Today, fewer than one million Assyrians remain in the Middle East. Over 100,000 Assyrians live in the United States, concentrated mainly in Chicago, Detroit, and Phoenix. There are over 70,000 Assyrians in Australia, including 40,000 in Sydney, an estimated 20,000 in Melbourne, and around 10,000 in the rest of Australia. There are around 100,000 Assyrians in Germany, 100,000 in Sweden, and around 10,000 in the UK.

There was a large influx of Assyrians into Australia in 2015, when the government agreed to a special intake of 18,563 refugees from Syria, the majority (80 per cent) of whom were Assyrians.

For further information, see UNPO (Unrepresented Nations and People's Organization) on the Assyrian diaspora.

Assyrian religion

Christianity took root amongst Aramaic-speaking Jews in Jerusalem and spread to other Aramaic-speaking Semitic peoples in Mesopotamia and along the Mediterranean coast in the 1st century AD. These early Assyrians, along with Armenians and Greeks, were amongst the first peoples to convert from polytheistic beliefs to Christianity, two centuries before Emperor Constantine promulgated Christianity as the religion of the Roman Empire. Organised Christian communities spread inland from the Mediterranean coast during the first three centuries AD and a literature of Syriac Christianity appeared.

Today, Assyrian Christianity is divided into several denominations: the Assyrian Catholic church, the Nestorian (Orthodox) Assyrian church, the Assyrian Chaldean church, and Protestant and evangelical churches.

Church ruins dating from the 3rd century provide evidence of the presence of organised Christian communities in the Aramaic-speaking area far inland from Jerusalem and the Mediterranean coast.

By the 4th century, an early literature of Syriac Christianity appeared. Aramaic speakers from Syria and Persia attended the first ecumenical council, known as The First Council of Nicaea, in 325 AD.

Tel Wardiyat

Tel Wardiyat is one of 30 villages that was established in north-east Syria for Assyrian refugees from Iraq, following the Simele massacre in 1933. The French, who were governing Syria at the time under the French Mandate, gained formal approval for the establishment of the Assyrian villages from the League of Nations. During the 1930s and 40s, around 20,000 Assyrians migrated from the region of Mosul in Iraq to escape the violence, establishing agricultural and business communities in the Hasakah region.

Since the beginning of the Syrian civil war in 2011, large numbers of Assyrians have emigrated from Tel Wardiyat and other Assyrian villages in the region, especially after attacks by ISIL in 2014 and 2015. ISIL was defeated in 2017 by the Kurdish and Syrian armies, but the villages are now largely empty of Assyrians, whose homes and lands have been occupied by local Kurdish people.

Cochineal

Cochineal is a red dye made from the dried, pulverised bodies of scale insects that live on cactus. It was first used a thousand years ago by the Aztec and Mayan peoples of North and Central America as a red dye for clothes. In the 16th century, cochineal was introduced into Europe where it was highly valued as a pigment in paints, a dye for fabrics, and a food colorant. Today, cochineal is imported mainly from Peru and the Canary Islands where the insects are grown on plantations of prickly pear cactus. The insects are sun-dried, crushed, and put into an acidic alcohol solution to produce carminic acid and cochineal extract.

Cochineal is not normally toxic but may provoke allergic reactions in some people.

What is braille?

The braille system of writing for visually impaired people was invented by Louis Braille, a Frenchman who lost his sight as the result of a childhood accident. In 1824, at the age of 15, he invented a code for the French alphabet based on small raised dots that are embossed on paper and can be read by touch. Today, braille writing can be printed by a computer with a braille embosser.

Braille characters take the form of rectangular blocks called cells, in which each letter of the alphabet is represented by a pattern of bumps. A full braille cell includes six raised dots arranged in two columns, each column having up to three dots. Each individual arrangement of up to six dots can be used to represent a letter, digit, punctuation mark, or word.

In English braille, there are three levels of encoding: Grade 1, a letter-by-letter transcription used for basic literacy. Grade 2 includes abbreviations and contractions. Grade 3, the highest level, can include various non-standardised combinations. Marie reads braille at the Grade 2 level.

Braille education is necessary for blind people to acquire literacy. However, in the face of changes in education policy and audio screen-reader software, braille usage has declined in recent decades, despite the fact that technologies such as braille displays have also made it more accessible and practical.

Digital communication technologies for visually impaired people

Since the last quarter of the 20th century, the digital revolution has transformed the way we all learn, work, and play. Accordingly, access to electronic communication has become necessary for equitable and effective participation in society by people who are blind.

Huge barriers, in the form of the graphical user interface using icons rather than text and the touchscreen used on smartphones, have presented major challenges.

The technical solution for the removal of these barriers is known as the screen-reader. Screen-reader software, which outputs in either synthetic speech or braille, enables a blind person to navigate a computer screen and to know the meaning of the icons and the textual information that is present. Synthetic speech refers to the technology of intelligible speech being created by a computer. Mainstream applications include satellite-based navigation systems used in cars, and virtual assistants such as Apple's Siri, Amazon's Alexa, and Google's Assistant.

While synthetic speech has underpinned mainstream applications in the 21st century, it has been used for much longer as the main computer-based access technology for blind people. Without synthetic speech, blind people would have been locked out of desk-based work and would have been seriously disadvantaged in access to high school and tertiary education, and to social media. It is reasonable, therefore, to conclude that synthetic speech is the most important development for effective participation in society by blind people since braille.

Helen Keller

Helen Adams Keller (1880–1968) became blind and deaf at the age of 19 months as the result of scarlet fever or meningitis. By the time she was six, without any means of communication, her behaviour had become wild and destructive. Her devoted parents were desperate to find a way of teaching her to communicate but were unable to control her raging tantrums.

Helen's parents sought advice from several experts and engaged 20-year-old Anne Sullivan as her teacher and companion. Anne had trained to work with deaf and blind children at the Perkins Institute for the Blind, in Boston, Massachusetts.

A brilliant, patient teacher, Anne calmed Helen's turbulent behaviour and eventually taught her to communicate with finger sign–language. After a long struggle, Helen learned to sign the letters of the alphabet, and she learned to copy Anne in signing words, but she still didn't understand the concept of a word, or the fact that everyday objects had names. She was unable to connect the patterns of finger signs with the objects that Anne was putting into her hands.

One day, Anne poured water on to her hand and spelled out the word 'water.' Suddenly, in great excitement, Helen tapped the same letters back into Anne's hand. She had finally grasped that there was a connection between objects and the finger signs that Anne tapped into her hands. She had discovered language: that things had names, and that people could communicate the names to each other. By the end of that day, she had learned to spell out the names of 30 objects — her first step towards education and what was to become a joyful and productive life.

Eventually, Helen learned to communicate ideas and feelings with finger sign–language, and to read and write in braille, read embossed print, and write letters with the aid of a writing frame.

Anne then taught Helen to 'hear' speech by placing her hand on the face of the speaker with her thumb on the larynx, her index finger on the lips, and her middle finger on the side of their nose. In that way, she could pick up the different facial movements and the different vibrations formed by vowels and consonants as they were spoken. Finally, Helen learned to speak by making sounds while reproducing the lip, mouth, and tongue movements in combination with the different vibrations. She often said that her greatest sadness was that she could not speak clearly enough for people to readily understand her. When Helen was giving her public lectures, Anne Sullivan had to translate her blurred speech into clearly audible speech.

In 1896, at the age of 16, Helen Keller enrolled in the Cambridge School for Young Ladies in Massachusetts, and by 1904, she was the first blind-deaf person to graduate from university with a Bachelor of Arts degree. In 1906, she published her famous memoir, *The Story of My Life,* which has been translated into 50 languages and has sold millions of copies worldwide. Helen wrote 12 books altogether, and published dozens of articles.

She became famous as a lecturer and advocate for social causes including the rights of blind and disabled people, universal education, women's suffrage, and workers' rights. She joined the Socialist Party, wrote a series of articles on socialism and world affairs entitled *Out of the Dark,* and spoke out on a range of issues. She testified before the American Congress on ways to improve the welfare of blind people, and was a tireless campaigner for blind people and other underprivileged groups.

Anne Sullivan married, and continued by Helen's side as her friend, carer, and teacher for almost 50 years. After she died in 1936, Polly Thomson, who had been Helen and Anne's secretary since 1914, took over Anne's role and remained by Helen's side for the next 24 years.

Between 1946 and 1957, Helen travelled to 35 different countries as a celebrated public lecturer and ambassador, speaking on behalf of blind and disabled people, women, and other disadvantaged groups. She met with American presidents from Franklin Roosevelt to Lyndon Johnson and dozens of world leaders. She was showered with awards, medals, and honorary doctoral degrees. In 1955, at age 75, she went on a 40,000-mile, five-month speaking trip across Asia, bringing inspiration and encouragement to millions.

Helen Keller died in 1968, at the age of 88, after suffering several strokes. Her life has been celebrated in books, films, TV documentaries, and a Broadway musical production. Her inspiration lives on.

Corneal transplants

The cornea is the transparent, dome-shaped outer layer of the eye in front of the black pupil and coloured iris. If corneas become diseased or scarred, they can be surgically removed and replaced with corneas taken from organ donors who have died. Corneal transplants have a 90 per cent success rate, and most patients who have corneal transplants can go home the same day or the day after. However, there is a low success rate for corneal transplants if patients also suffer from glaucoma or some other eye disease.

Glaucoma

Glaucoma is the leading cause of blindness worldwide. Approximately 300,000 Australians have glaucoma, and 50 per cent of people with glaucoma go undiagnosed. One in eight Australians over the age of 80 will develop glaucoma.

Glaucoma affects the optic nerve connecting the eye to the brain. It is usually caused by a build-up of pressure in the eyeball ('high intraocular pressure') as the result of a blockage in the eye's drainage system.

Glaucoma can be treated with medication, laser treatment, or surgery, but there is currently no lasting cure.

Congenital or *infantile* glaucoma is distinguished from the primary glaucoma that normally affects around 1 per cent of the population worldwide. Congenital glaucoma is a rare condition caused by the defective development of the eye's drainage system *before* birth.

Early symptoms include enlarged eyes, increased tearing, sensitivity to light, and cloudiness of the cornea.

Medical treatments may involve surgery, the use of topical eye drops, and oral medications. These treatments help to either increase the exit of fluid from the eye or decrease the production of fluid inside the eye.

Congenital glaucoma affects approximately 1 in 10,000 people. Its frequency is higher in the Middle East.

The Royal Victorian Institute for the Blind

In 1866, the Victorian Asylum and School for the Blind was established as a refuge for blind, homeless, and sick people, especially children, who roamed the streets of Melbourne during the gold rush era. In 1868, the Asylum moved into a stately, purpose-built bluestone building in St Kilda Road, funded by a government grant and charitable subscriptions from the newly wealthy middle classes. Inmates, as they were known at the time, were given accommodation and training, establishing industries in basket-weaving, woodwork, net-making, brush-making, and knitting.

By January 1877, there were 103 inmates in the Asylum and School for the Blind, ranging in age between eight and 55 years old. Conditions were poor, with 40 or so people working and sleeping in large dormitories in a cold stone building with little or no heating. Inmates worked to both pay for their keep and to make an income for the asylum. Girls scrubbed the floors and did the laundry. Some trained as musicians and singers who went on tour around the state, giving concerts that earned the Asylum hundreds of pounds.

In 1891, the organisation was renamed the Royal

Victorian Institute for the Blind (RVIB). In the decades leading up to the 1920s, the inmates were often harshly treated, with forced labour for six days a week and corporal punishment for those who rebelled. Over the following decades, the RVIB developed enlightened and more humane policies, offering social and educational opportunities, including the teaching of braille, medical and ophthalmological care, and operations to restore sight. A new school was built and a braille library was established to produce and provide books in braille.

During the Second World War, the school buildings of the RVIB were acquired by the Commonwealth Government for use by the army. The children were moved from St Kilda to a holiday resort in Olinda, called 'The Georgian'. There they enjoyed the freedom of the bush surrounds and more independence than they had ever before known, remembered as 'a time of liberation and happiness'.

By the late 1990s, the RVIB became increasingly decentralised and offered a wide range of services to clients including mobility, occupational therapy, braille instruction, adaptive technologies, volunteer co-ordination, audio books and magazines, radio for the Print Handicapped (3RPH), and supported employment.

In 2004, the RVIB merged with other organisations around Australia to form Vision Australia. The heritage-listed building on St Kilda Road is now a commercial venue and boutique hotel.

For further information on the history of the RVIB, see Buckrich, J R. (2004). *Lighthouse on the Boulevard: A History of the Royal Victorian Institute for the Blind.* Australian Scholarly Publishing, Melbourne.

The Migrant Women's Learning Centre (MWLC)

The Migrant Women's Learning Centre (MWLC) was started by Lella Fazzalori as a shop-front community-education program in Collingwood in the 1980s, based on the existing Footscray Women's Learning Centre. At the time Marie studied there, in the early 90s, the MWLC was part of the Language Studies Department of what was first Collingwood TAFE (Technical and Further Education College), then part of the Northern Metropolitan College of TAFE (NMCOT), later North Melbourne Institute of Technology (NMIT), and now Melbourne Polytechnic. Physically, the MWLC occupied old technical-school buildings on Johnston St and then Wellington St.

In 1990, Miriam Faine became the Co-ordinator of the MWLC. From this time, the Centre developed a unique adult English as a Second Language (ESL) program that responded to women ESL learners' levels of language attainment and general education as well as their personal needs, such as childcare, in order to situate their English language learning within the context of their lived experience. This program was based on the understanding that language and literacy are social practices that are best taught, from the earliest stages, alongside and through vocational training and basic education. Overall, the MWLC's philosophy was to move away from the framing of immigrant women as people who needed helping.

The social relations and practices underlying the MWLC were embedded in its pedagogy, organisational structures, and even the physical facilities. The Centre organised functions or parties at the end of each semester that featured performances, or exhibitions, or prominent speakers, as well as dancing and food. There were regular presentations from community health workers and other organisations working with immigrant women. Films and excursions were part of the curriculum. These also had a social function, and brought all the students together so that women could meet students from other classes and make friends who spoke the same language[s]. It was particularly important to introduce the less privileged and more isolated women to accessible recreational facilities: often, they had never visited the city or the Yarra parks a few kilometres away. Similarly, each semester ended with a trip to the bush or the beach — new experiences for some of the students.

The Centre operated as a 'women's only' space. For example, most of the women who covered their hair would take their hijab off once inside. This signified the integrity of the Centre as a separate space. Kitchen facilities and a microwave were provided, together with a central lounge area. The physical environment of the Centre was also a learning environment: maps, posters, and notice boards lined the walls. Bookshelves contained a collection of bilingual dictionaries and English dictionaries, atlases and other reference materials, a small collection of books in English, and also the discards from the local library's community-language collection (Barbara Cartland in Turkish, for example).

Many women preferred women's only provision. Some curriculum areas like Women's Health would have been impossible to study in a mixed class. Other discussions about personal relationships would have been difficult, or different. For example, some of the students were recovering from abusive relationships. The commonality of women's experiences across ethnic groups, and even between teachers and students, was stressed over and over again.

From the Centre's beginning, the larger number of prospective students came from poor backgrounds, and many had had little or even no formal schooling, requiring an explicit focus on literacy in the ESL teaching. While most of the students wanted to learn English to find a job, this translated into improving literacy, understood as encompassing learning many other things about the world, like geography, science, and maths — what is often called adult basic education.

The Centre, then, was a space within which immigrant women like Marie had the opportunity to reposition themselves, as confident users of Australian English, as employable, and as 'educated'.

Vision Australia

Vision Australia is the national provider of services to Australians who are blind or have low vision. The organisation was formed in 2004 through the merger of the Vision Australia Foundation, the Royal Victorian Institute for the Blind, and the Royal Blind Society of NSW. In 2008, the Royal Blind Foundation Queensland

and Seeing Eye Dogs Australia also merged with Vision Australia.

Vision Australia estimates that there are approximately 357,000 people who are blind or vision impaired currently living in Australia, with more than 70 per cent over the age of 65. More than 25,000 Australians who are visually disabled receive support from Vision Australia, including more than 3,000 children. A wide range of client-based services are offered to support and assist people to live the life they choose. These services include: seeing-eye dogs; a large braille, talking book, and digital library; a network of ten radio stations for people with print handicaps; a range of accessible technology for sale through retail stores; training in the use of accessible technology; occupational therapy, orientation, and mobility instruction, counselling, and physiotherapy.

Vision Australia relies on government funding as well as donations from philanthropic trusts and foundations, bequests, and money raised by local clubs, committees, and auxiliaries. For more than 80 years, thousands of people have flocked to Vision Australia's major fund-raising event, 'Carols by Candlelight', which is held in the Sidney Myer Music Bowl on Christmas Eve.

Thousands of volunteers contribute their time and skills to Vision Australia or directly to clients.

Foundation House — the Victorian Foundation for the Survivors of Torture Inc.

Foundation House exists to support the mental health, well-being, and rights of people from refugee backgrounds, many of whom have experienced torture or other traumatic events in their countries of origin.

With its head office in Gardiner Street, Brunswick, Foundation House provides services in Dallas (Broadmeadows), Dandenong, Ringwood, and Sunshine, and supports a network of professional staff in through agencies in rural and regional Victoria.

Each year, Foundation House provides services to more than 5,000 people from refugee backgrounds. Since 1987, it has supported and empowered thousands of survivors of torture and other traumatic experiences to rebuild their lives. It advocates to government and other agencies for policies and services to promote well-being of refugees and asylum seekers and conducts research to improve access to services.

Its staff of approximately 200 people includes psychiatrists, psychologists, counsellors, social workers, interpreters, and professionals in the fields of community development, health promotion, natural therapies, management, finance, information technology, and administration. Their approach is to work with an understanding of survivors' individual histories, their current problems, and the supports and opportunities available in Australia.

Red Cross Volunteer Service

There are several hundred Red Cross volunteers around Australia who provide direct help and support to disabled people. Marie wishes to thank the volunteer drivers who for five years drove her the 30-odd kilometres from her home in Reservoir to the RVIB in St Kilda and back, two or three days a week. She always enjoyed being picked up and driven by friendly Red Cross drivers who made her attendance at the RVIB possible.

Diploma of Interpreting (LOTE — English)

The Diploma of Interpreting offered by the Royal Melbourne Institute of Technology is a one-year full-time course that qualifies bilingual people for careers in professional interpreting. Students are trained to retain words spoken in one language and reproduce them in another language. Learning activities include lectures, tutorials, simulations, case studies, role plays, group discussions, and practical demonstrations. At the time of writing, the course is offered for interpretation between English and seven other languages spoken in Melbourne's multilingual communities.

Acknowledgements

I thank my family for the love and encouragement that has enabled me to write this book. My Melbourne brother and sisters — Younan, Antoinette, Sherine, Janet, Hanne, Margaret, and their families — have supported and shared memories. My American sisters, Nimo, Mona, and Rima, are always there on the end of the phone, asking me about the book and encouraging me. My nieces and nephews always say, 'Hurry up and finish your book — we can't wait to read it!'

Ivan Molloy, who connected me with services for blind people when I first came to Melbourne, is one of my oldest Australian friends. I thank him and his wife, Lorraine, for inviting us to their home and telling us stories about the RVIB and Ben Hewitt in the old days.

I thank my Australian friends, especially my Migrant

Women's Learning Centre friends Veronica, Lorraine, and the teachers for their friendship over the years and for meeting with us to talk about our MWLC years.

I thank Jacob Haweil of the Australian Assyrian Arts and Literature Foundation for his Assyrian-language radio program and for giving us information about the Assyrian community in Australia.

Thanks to friends and colleagues at Foundation House who have given me interest and encouragement, and thanks to its CEO, Paris Aristotle, for his input.

I especially thank Bill Jolley for his enthusiastic feedback, his help, and for his lovely words in the foreword of this book. Thanks to Steve Jolley for his encouragement, and his years as presenter on 3RPH (Radio Print Handicapped — now Radio Vision Australia), which I love listening to. Thanks to Ron Hooton, CEO of Vision Australia, for his support and assistance. I thank Vision Australia for all the wonderful work they do for blind people; I especially appreciate the talking-book library, where I can get any information I need.

A big thank you to all the people at Scribe for all they have done to make the book a reality. I'm so proud of it.

I could never have written this book without my teacher, friend, and co-author Jill Sanguinetti. Thank you, Jill, for all your hard work putting the stories of my life together and writing them into a book. You made my words sound better and my story more interesting. I feel as if I cooked a plain meal, and then you put in the right spices to bring out the taste of the food so people would want to eat it, and turn to the next page, and the next. David was always there with good ideas and support. I can't thank you both enough.

Marie Younan

Thanks to all my friends who have read bits of this book along the way and given feedback, especially Nick Legge, Delia Bradshaw, Jane Loudon, Rosemary Ingram, and Michael O'Donnell. Thanks to John Jenkins for warm encouragement and for doing an early edit of the manuscript.

Thanks to my Migrant Women's Learning Centre mates, especially Miriam Faine and Elizabeth Connell, for keeping in contact over the years and feeding their memories in.

Bill Jolley and Stephen Jolley were the first blind people to read the book. Their appreciation of Marie's journey and their role in bringing the book to the attention of Vision Australia has been pivotal. Thanks to

Ron Hooton, CEO of Vision Australia, for his input and the offer of Vision Australia's support in promoting the print and audio versions.

My sister Margot Rosenbloom, who is a Scribe editor, gave me the invaluable advice several years ago to 'just keep on writing' through the messy stages. I thank her and Scribe's founder and publisher, Henry Rosenbloom, for believing in our book and taking it on as a Scribe publication. Thanks to all the Scribe team, especially associate publisher Marika Webb-Pullman and managing editor Kevin O'Brien for warm and productive collaborations under lockdown. Thanks to Guy Ivison for his beautiful book and cover design.

Thank you, David Legge: my dear partner, editor extraordinaire, computer nerd, and trusty source of ideas, information, support, and laughter. Marie and I would not have been able to complete our book without you.

And Marie: thank you for trusting me with your story, and for all I have learned in the telling and writing of it.

Jill Sanguinetti